CHAIR YOGA FOR SENIORS

Guided Exercises for Elderly to Improve Balance, Flexibility and Increase Strength After 60

BAZ THOMPSON

CONTENTS

BEFORE YOU START READING

As a special gift, I included a logbook and my book, **"Strength Training After 40"** (regularly priced at $16.97 on Amazon) and the best part is, you get access to all of them.

FREE

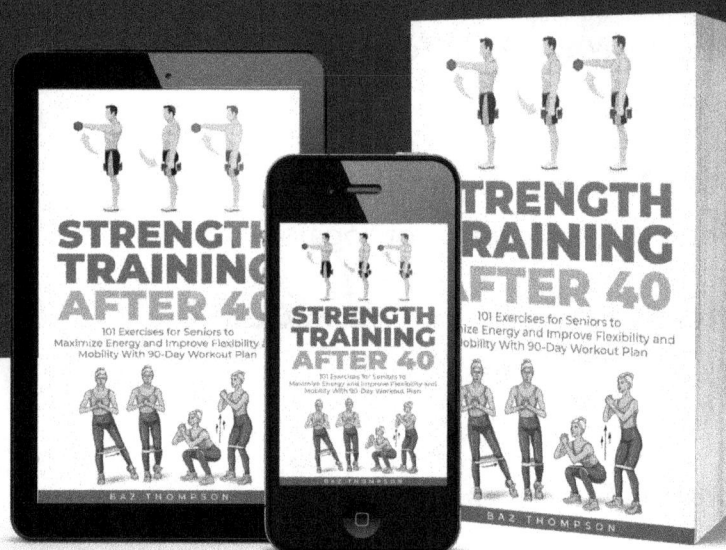

WHAT'S IN IT FOR ME?

- 101 highly effective strength training exercises that can help you reach the highest point of your fitness performance

- Foundational exercises to improve posture and increase range of motion in your arms, shoulders, chest, and back

- Stretches to help you gain flexibility and find deep relaxation

- Workout Logbook to help you keep track of your accomplishments and progress. Log your progress to give you the edge you need to accomplish your goals.

SCAN ME

INTRODUCTION

There is an unsaid puzzle surrounding growing old. It is said that to stay healthy and well one has to be active, but to stay active, one has to have a body that allows this. If throwing Frisbees or playing soccer won't do, what can we do to live a healthy lifestyle? Sir Michael Marmot, in his book, The Health Gap, introduces an important concept. One that aging people everywhere intuitively understand: living a life that is worthwhile. The concept is simple: living to a hundred years is not desirable if you are going to spend the majority of that time ill and unable to enjoy your life. More years added to your life is only desirable if it means you can also enjoy that life just as well as your fifties, for example. The way to do that is by staying agile and eating well. The eating part is simple enough but staying active seems to become more difficult with age.

The sad news is that a great deal of us don't have bodies that can do strenuous exercises. There are some of us confined to wheelchairs or have limited mobility at any age. So, if someone were to suggest yoga as a solution, it would seem strange. After all, yoga demands a certain kind of flexibility and strength that many of us don't possess as we mature, especially if we're never active.

However, yoga is a more accessible solution for many people. If only there was a way to do yoga without subjecting our bodies to extremes. Herein comes chair yoga. Chair yoga can help increase flexibility, strength and offers benefits of active exercise without subjecting our bodies to harm. Turns out there is a way to live a life that is worthwhile after all. That is what this book is ultimately about, allowing you to live the full life you deserve in your golden years. Chair yoga, paired with eating well and other healthy habits, is an excellent way to accomplish that.

Here's how the book is structured. We will spend the first and second chapters looking at yoga and how it applies to your situation and what you can expect to gain from it. In the third and fourth chapters, we will introduce exercises designed to help you live a life that is worthwhile. In the fifth and final chapters, we will introduce yoga routines you can practice every day to improve strength, balance, and flexibility.

Please accept my deepest thanks for reading my book. Please let me know what you think by leaving a review on Amazon. This will help a lot of other people who are also looking for a book like mine. That would be extremely beneficial to me.

Scan the QR Code To Leave a Review:

My hope and desire is that you will find this book useful as you strive to regain and maintain good balance in order to prevent falls and enhance your overall well-being.

Here's to a better you!

Chapter 1

WHY CHAIR YOGA

Chair yoga is trauma informed, meaning it is created with challenges in mind. The aim is to make it as easy as possible for anyone interested in yoga. We want you to try it, regardless of your history. Yoga is one of the most well-suited activities for seniors because of how gentle it is while offering many of the benefits associated with traditional exercises.

In the U.S., when you reach the age of 65, you can expect to live for another 15 years or more (Pfau, 2016). Whether you enjoy those years depends on how you choose to live. If you opt to be less active, you risk worsening many of the conditions that tend to inflict seniors. Being active is the sure way to ensure you enjoy your retirement years.

The leading causes of death among seniors are heart disease, cancer, chronic lower respiratory disease and stroke (Heron, 2021). It's no secret that as we age, we become less flexible. It can be from growing old and from conditions that tend to afflict seniors. Conditions like osteoarthritis and rheumatoid arthritis can decrease our flexibility. Through life we accumulate injuries that leave a mark. The river life has a way of sculpting, marking and eroding the body, if we stay still, the river of life is merciless. Thankfully, we can do something to lessen its impact and improve our happiness.

BENEFITS OF YOGA

Many seniors suffer from other chronic illnesses that can affect their quality of life. If you're going to live a long life, you want it to be enjoyable. Choosing an activity like chair yoga is one way to go about it. Why? It's safe, effective, and enjoyable. Plus, it's cheap and you can do it anywhere.

Chair yoga improves one's balance, mobility, and flexibility, something that many seniors lose as they age. This minimizes the chance of injury as a result of losing balance or from a lack of flexibility. As a senior, you may begin to accept that being inflexible is just a part of the deal but it doesn't have to be the case.

Frequent aches and pains, whether from disease, or from age are common among seniors. They experience joint pain, inflammation in the fingers, hips, spine and more. Yoga has been shown to ease pain and the discomfort that comes from swollen, tender joints or arthritis symptoms.

A stereotype of someone who does yoga often is of someone who is calm and at peace. That characterization is not so bad because yoga reduces stress and promotes mental wellness. These can help with high blood pressure which is a contributing factor to heart disease. The relaxation that happens as a result of yoga helps us sleep better. Sleep is integral to almost any part of our health. As we age, sleep quality and quantity decrease which is bad for many of our health systems.

Just how important is sleep? It's imperative for your immune system, for brain function, our heart, memory, learning and body weight. A lack of sleep has been linked to a higher risk of medical conditions like: obesity, type 2 diabetes, high blood pressure, heart disease, stroke, poor mental health, safe driving, mood, and early death (Pacheco, 2020).

Research has shown that the brains of people with Alzheimer's struggle with achieving the quality of sleep needed for the proper function of the brain. This might explain why quality sleep, (achieved through intervention) can improve those symptoms or even delay the onset of Alzheimer's or similar diseases (Walker, 2019).

As we grow older, our quality of sleep tends to decline. A lack of sleep affects our cognitive performance, which explains why forgetfulness and other diseases affecting cognition are common in older people.

Yoga will help you develop a strong core. A strong core is especially good for seniors and those with limited mobility because it helps us avoid injuries. It also helps with back pain, digestion, and breathing. It's very important for seniors to maintain independence, carry out their daily tasks with ease, engage in leisure activities and maintain good posture. All things that a healthy core is integral to (Webster, 2018).

When you add all of this up, you have a very confident person whose mood is improved and feels healthier. That makes us happier. It's so empowering. You want that. It's a motivating feeling, as if you can do anything. It's especially desirable at an age where many fear of losing their autonomy. It's good to gain it back.

KEY TAKEAWAY

I like saying that chair yoga will help clients get their life back. It's not an exaggeration because the benefits from chair yoga set off a chain reaction of positive outcomes that improve the quality of your life overall. Your golden years can be filled with less pain, sickness and discomfort. You can remain active, autonomous, sharp, and healthy for longer. If you have lost your spark, it can help you regain it.

Chapter 2

DOING YOGA THE RIGHT WAY

To do yoga properly and reap some of the benefits from the previous chapter, there are some habits and techniques you will have to adopt. These will allow us to get the best out of our yoga exercises. They apply across all of the yoga exercises we will cover in this book and beyond. Always be safe and follow the instructions.

GETTING THE MOST OUT OF YOGA

First, respect the limits of your body. Never overextend. Make sure that you are always feeling comfortable and stable in whatever exercise you do. If you push things too far too quickly, you could harm yourself, so be careful.

Improvement will happen on its own, slowly but surely. There's no need to rush things. A good way to tell if you are taking things a bit far is by paying attention to your facial expressions. If you're finding yourself grimacing, that might be a sign that you are pushing things a little bit further than you can handle.

Second, pay attention to your breathing. In yoga, breathing is everything. It helps center the mind and is also good for facilitating yoga. Let's talk about why that is. Breathing will help calm your muscles, lower blood pressure and improve circulation, meaning different organs get the oxygen that they need to perform at their peak and avoid injury. The prevention of injury is important in trauma informed yoga practice (Southard, 2019).

Breathing also helps with meditation and mood. For yoga, happiness and mediation are important, especially when you want all the benefits we explored in the previous chapter. Yoga is not just a form of exercise. Yoga is also a form of meditation. It is a blend of the physical and the mental which makes it the perfect exercise because it provides the physical benefits of exercise and meditation in one activity. This is one of the reasons why it's so powerful and popular with people of all ages (Southard, 2019).

Lastly, make sure you are fully hydrated before and after a yoga session. This is important for injury prevention and improving movement. Also, having to stop a session to get a glass of water can interrupt your flow, which is essential for the meditative aspect of yoga.

Common Mistakes

Good yoga practice is also about knowing what not to do. The tips in this section are also about avoiding bad habits that may lead to undesirable consequences (Jones, 2019).

Trying Too Hard

Because yoga is understood as an exercise, many people believe that they have to do it 'hard' to reap the benefits of it. This is fine when you want to build muscle by lifting weights but with yoga that sort of mentality is not necessary. Yoga is also about being deliberate and delicate in how you conduct yourself. Here relaxation is not a bad thing. So, if you experience pain or discomfort, it is not necessarily a

sign you are doing something right. Often it is a sign you are pushing too hard. So, take it easy. This is even more important with seniors.

Eating Before Yoga

It is best not to eat right before yoga so that you can allow blood to be in another place in your body instead of busy digesting the food.. With other kinds of strenuous exercise, it may be advised to eat first to help give your body the fuel it needs to get through tough exercises. With yoga, you are not going to be doing anything too strenuous, so it does not make sense to do this. You need parts of your body to have enough resources to move freely, which is harder after having eaten.

Rushing Through Stages

Avoid going for advanced exercises when you are beginning and focus on mastering the basics. Most of what we will do will be the basics and that is for good reason. When your foundations are off, taking on more advanced routines will either not give you the benefit you are looking for or, in the worst case, injure you.

Obsessing Too Much Over Form

Many people, when they start yoga, want to achieve perfect form. That might mean they push themselves too hard to achieve the right form. Instead, your focus should be on the little progress you are making. The perfect form will come with time and practice. Also focus on progress, be gentle and patient.

Not Warming Up

I know warming up can seem like a waste. It may appear indulgent, boring and even pointless. But you need to warm up to ready your mind and body for the session. Warmups are a key ingredient for a successful session of yoga, so don't skip them. A key component of that is also the warm down.

Not Understanding the Difference Between Good and Bad Pain

With any type of exercise there will be some pain and discomfort. Some of that pain is a good sign (like we are awakening the right muscles) and some of it is bad (like we are damaging some muscles). Because pain is subjective , it is hard for people to know if the pain they are experiencing is the right kind of pain or the bad kind of pain. Some people believe, erroneously, that the worse the pain the better, that it shows that they are making more progress.

Understand this: pain is the body's way of telling us something is damaged, will become damaged or is being damaged. The qualities of these types of pain are different. Bad pain tells you something is damaged. It is restrictive and very uncomfortable. It is your body screaming, stop this now! Good pain is your body telling you to be careful, to take it easy. It is often experienced as mild discomfort, there is nothing sharp and acute about it.

You need to listen to your body. Your body's inner voice is soft and curious when you raise your arms. That is good. If it starts raising its voice when you raise your arms, maybe you should stop before that turns into a scream. You need to pay close attention to the inner voice. Remember to pay attention to the muscles in your face. If the pain is causing you to grimace that is a sign you should pull things back a little.

KEY
TAKEAWAY

Doing yoga is more than an exercise, it's a form of meditation, meaning pushing yourself is not always the best idea. You need to take your time, be gentle, keep hydrated and never forget the importance of breathing.

Chapter 3

WARM-UPS & WARM DOWNS

We talked about warm-ups and warm downs as being an important part of a successful yoga routine. In this chapter we will explore basic warm-up and warm down exercises. We will finish up with a routine that includes them both, that you can integrate later. Warm-ups can be used as warm downs, so there won't be two sections devoted to each in this chapter.

That means a typical yoga routine looks like this: warm-up, yoga exercises and then a warm down. The warm-up and warm down are always almost identical, just like typical athletic exercises. Another thing about warm-ups is that they can feel like a mini yoga in themselves.

I will begin this chapter by focusing on breathing exercises. The reasoning for this is simple: breathing exercises are a good way to transition from living life and into a session. The beauty of them is that they stimulate the mediation part of yoga and help relax the body. The breathing exercises themselves are not the warm-up, they are the build-up to a warm-up routine.

BREATHING EXERCISES

We are going to do two kinds of breathing exercises. They are the safest for beginners and people who may have limited mobility. Apart from that, they are just really good. I will begin by detailing what the exercise looks like and then describe how you would do it, followed by an example of the complete exercise.

Three Point Breathing

The three-point breathing is about breathing into three points of your body and exhaling from those too, in an ordered manner. When you inhale you have to imagine you are filling your belly, then your ribs and then your chest. When you exhale you have to exhale from the chest, ribs and then the belly. Just exhaling in reverse order of your inhale.

First you need a sturdy chair with good back support. When you are seated in the chair your feet should be able to touch the floor and your legs fold as close to a right angle as possible. Preferably the chair should not have arms, but if it does make sure there is enough space for you to move your arms to the side. You should not use rockers, swivel chairs or deep lounge seats. Dining chairs and similar chairs will work great.

Sit in the chair and place your hands on your thighs towards your knees. Ensure that you are not leaning on the back rest, and your posture is straight. Don't force things, if your posture doesn't allow you to be completely up straight, sit how you are most comfortable. Your palms may face up if you prefer. Now, relax your shoulders and close your eyes. Make sure your arms are relaxed as well.

1. Inhale deeply and then exhale. This is to prepare yourself.

2. Now, inhale into your lower belly. Hold your breath for two or three seconds and exhale. You can inhale through the nose and exhale through the mouth, do it the other way around or just stick with what feels natural to you. When inhaling into your belly you should feel the belly expand.

3. Inhale into your belly, hold for about a second and inhale into your ribs, just above your upper stomach. Hold for two or three seconds. Exhale the air from your ribs, hold, and then exhale air from your belly. When inhaling into the ribs you should fill pressure just below your rib cage.

4. Inhale into your belly, then hold. Inhale into your ribs then hold. Inhale into your chest and hold for two or three seconds. Exhale the air in your chest, hold. Exhale the air from your ribs, hold, then exhale the air from your belly. When inhaling into your chest you should feel pressure in your chest.

5. Repeat step four once.

6. Inhale into your belly and ribs and then exhale from your ribs followed by your belly. Step similar to step three.

7. Inhale into your belly and exhale after holding for two or three seconds. This is similar to step two.

8. Inhale then exhale. This is the first step, completing a round.

When I say hold without specifying the number of seconds, I just mean hold for about half-second to a second in between the different stages. The idea behind this exercise is to help you learn how to control your breathing. You will be doing a lot of controlled breathing in your yoga routines. Three-point breathing can be repeated for three rounds or more rounds before you move on to other parts of your routine. If you feel like a round is enough, and you are feeling a bit tired, take a break between rounds. Just do slow, comfortable breathing, with eyes closed and keep focusing on your breathing.

Alternate Nostril Breathing

You can include this alternate nostril breathing after three-point breathing, as it is very good at calming the central nervous system. If you find three-point breathing difficult you can just do alternate nostril breathing alone. Once you are comfortable with controlling your breathing you can then give three-point breathing a shot again. Alternate nostril breathing is the easiest of the two and it forces us to focus on our breathing a little more as breathing is paired with action.

Before you begin, make sure you are seated upright and you should be relaxed, in the chair of your choosing. For this exercise, eyes may be open.

1. Use your index finger and your middle finger to plug your right-hand side nostril. Don't put the fingers in your nostril, just apply pressure on the nostril, from the outside, to plug it.

2. Inhale through the left nostril.

3. Hold your breath for a second.

4. Plug your left nostril and exhale through you right nostril

5. With your hand still plugging your left nostril. Inhale through the right nostril.

6. Hold your breath for 2 seconds.

7. Plug your right nostril and exhale through the left nostril.

8. Repeat the process again.

As you go on, hold your breathing a little longer. You can do rounds like these for five minutes or more.

WARM-UP ROUTINE

Sit with your spine away from the back of the chair and feet planted on the floor, legs bending at 90-degree angle. This is called the seated mountain pose. Draw your hands to your chest, right in the middle, connecting your palms in what looks like prayer hands. Relax your shoulders and push your hands together, not too hard. You just want them to lightly touch. Pushing them together too hard may hurt your wrists, don't lift your elbows too high as that may contribute to the stress in your wrists.

Then you slowly drop your hands towards your lap, down the center. As you get close to your lap, you begin to inhale and then sweep up your hands in wide arcs from the sides. You lift your hands up above your head where you connect them together again and then exhale. As you sweep up your hands make sure. Drop your hand to your chest again and repeat the exercise again, dropping your hand to your hands towards your lap as you inhale and sweep. Exhaling right above your head when your hand connects again.

Next rest your hands on your knees and circle your shoulders forward. Do these five to six times, remembering to stay relaxed. Then reverse by rotating your shoulders backwards. Do it for the same amount of time. Stay loose and don't do it too quickly or too slowly. Your shoulders feel a little funny if you are not used to doing this; that is fine, it's nothing to worry about.

Then you will transition to neck circles. When doing neck circles, you shouldn't aim to do a full rotation of the neck yet. Just slowly rotate your neck to one shoulder and slowly drop at the center, neck touching the chest if you can, and then rise up to the shoulder on the other side. Put your shoulders down and relax as you do it. Repeat the same motion from side to side three to five times, then drop at the center and raise your head to normal.

Lift hands a little and slowly roll the wrists. Be slow and careful as not to injure yourself. Don't bend the wrists too much if it causes you pain. Just roll them nicely and slowly in a way that is comfortable for you.

Then you will do the same thing with your ankles. If you can, lift your legs up slightly and give your ankles roll. Then try stretching out your toes. Again, if movement is very uncomfortable don't force it and keep things smooth and natural feeling. If you lift your legs too high you will tire quickly, so a light lift is mandatory. We don't want to test your leg muscles with this one. Do two or three rotations and then ground your feet.

We are now going to do a side bend. To do this use one of your hands to grab the seat. This hand will work as your support. Inhale, sweeping up your free hand in a wide arch and bend towards your side with your free hand reaching to the side you are bending towards as if reaching for something.

Then, bend the elbow of the arm that is reaching over the side. Exhale as you bend the elbow. Remember to keep the arm up and over your head as you do this. When you bend your elbow your hand should draw to the other side of your head. Inhale as you reach to the side and exhale each time you bend your elbow. Do this two to three times,

Now go back to the center, connect your hands and repeat the same exercise, this time on the other side. Make sure the number of times you do it is equal.

If you would rather not grab the side of your chair for support to do this exercise, you can just let your other arm hang free if you are confident in your ability to balance. I advised you to hold the chair so you can avoid falling and injury. Sweep up your arms together one more time, inhaling. Exhale, and rest your hands on your knees or close.

Now, begin circling from the waist. Going forward, to the side, back, side and front again. Keep circling for two or three rotations before reversing (anti-clockwise and clockwise, do equal rotations).

Now, claim your center again and then scoot forward in your chair, arching in the front. Make sure your chest comes forward while your back dips. Don't force it and do it to the extent it feels comfortable. This is called the cow pose. Hold it a little and then arch your back like a cat, making sure your chest falls in. Alternate between the two poses a couple of times before returning to the center again.

Let's repeat the same poses again but inhaling when we march forward in the cow pose and exhaling when we arch our backs and chest falls like a cat. Put your legs apart so that you can arch forward again, lifting your heart but this time a little harder and past your shoulders, inhale while you do it. Then drop your chest and arch your back making sure your heart drops behind your shoulders and exhales. Make sure your spine presses back as you exhale, to make sure you are getting the pose right.

Now, sit back up straight and sweep up your hands, inhaling as you do and then exhale as you bring your hands back down to your knees.

That concludes the warm-up exercise.

What you do is begin with both or one of the breathing exercises and then transition into this routine. After you are done with the routine you can then do some of the exercises we will share in the coming chapters. Please, don't skip the warm-up and remember to warm-down with this routine after you have done your core yoga routine. It is super important!

KEY TAKEAWAY

The routines in here can be used as a warm down and warm up. Alternatively, and I did not mention this, you can use them as a routine in and of themselves. Warm ups will help lessen and prevent injuries during the bigger and longer yoga sessions.

Chapter 4
EXERCISES

In these sections we will explore some chair yoga exercises. These exercises can be performed alone or as part of a yoga routine. Many of these are simple and foundational, and that is with purpose. Many of the poses and stretches in this section form the basis for many yoga routines. It is helpful to think of the exercises in this section as ingredients for a recipe. They can be put together to make yoga routines. In that sense, if you want, you can make your own yoga routine by combining these exercises.

Getting these exercises right and knowing them is crucial. As an added benefit, many of these exercises are very versatile. They can be performed almost anywhere, and at any time with very little set up. I have used them at various down time moments throughout my days for the benefits they offer.

These exercises are good for releasing energy, relieving tension, dealing with pain, helping with flexibility and improving mood. If you are not active at all, you will feel them in your body. You will feel those aches that come with activating your muscles the first time or using them in new ways. Remember that this is a good type of pain. You will begin to feel yourself become firmer in some areas, more flexible, responsive, balanced and experience less pain overall.

Before we go into it, some causation is warranted. Before you take part in any of these exercises, especially if you have a condition you think may be worsened by some exercise, consult your doctor. Otherwise, proceed with caution. Exercises in these sections are safe and simple, but I can't account for every situation out there when putting them together. If something doesn't feel right, don't push.

LOWER
BODY

The exercises below are targeted at the lower body. If you have foot or leg problems, the exercises in this section may help with swelling, pain and help strengthen the leg muscles.

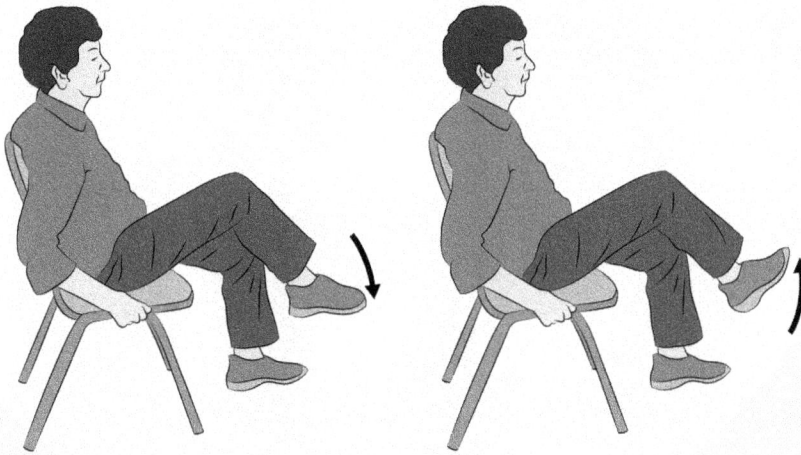

FOOT CIRCLES

DURATION: 2 TO 5 MINUTES

Foot circles, like we have done in our warm-up routines, are good for enhancing mobility and relieving tension. They also strengthen the muscles in front of our shins. You can also do this exercise after a long day standing up or using your feet.

HOW TO

1. Sit in a standard mountain pose. This means sitting tall and straight, with legs slightly apart, hands on your knees and shoulders behind your ears. Make sure your legs are bent at the knees at a 90 degree angle. Relax.

2. Raise your right foot as high as you can but never above your seat. Then circle your right foot counterclockwise ten times and repeat clockwise. As you do this, breathe slowly.

3. Put your right foot down to assume the mountain pose again. Take a few deep breaths and repeat the same exercise on your left foot.

4. You can repeat this as long as you feel comfortable before moving to other exercises.

5. To finish the exercise off, and only if you feel comfortable and capable, do both feet at the same time.

Step five is not a must, but you should try it when you have gone through the exercise plenty and you feel you could use a little more challenge.

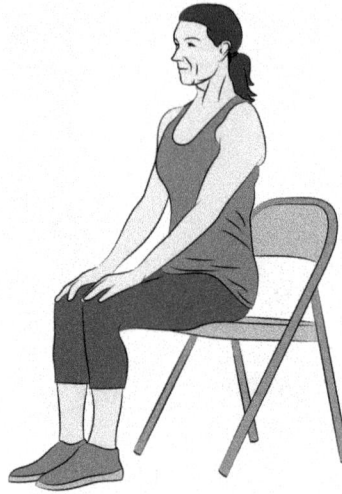

BUTT SQUEEZE

DURATION: 1 TO 3 MINUTES

Butt squeezes are good at working pelvic floor muscles, buttocks and inner thighs.

HOW TO

1. To begin, sit with your feet hip-width and with hips towards the edge of the chair and hands on your knees.

2. Now, squeeze your buttocks together as if you are going to stand up. Hold the squeeze for two to three seconds and release.

3. Repeat these squeezes twenty or more times. You can do this for a couple of more sets if you wish.

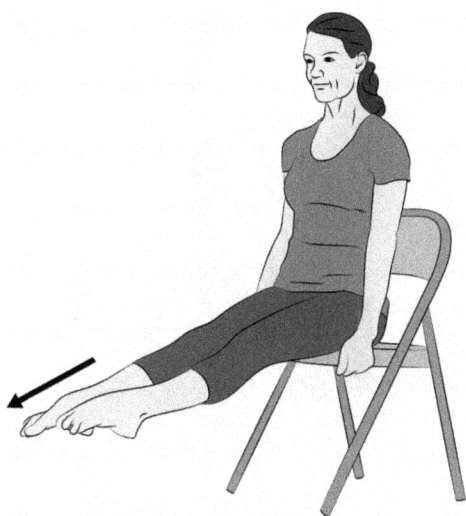

POINT AND FLEX

DURATION: 2 TO 4 MINUTES

With this exercise we hope to make your feet and ankles more flexible. It's also good for anyone who wears very restrictive shoes. Your calf muscles and shins will be worked as well when doing this exercise.

HOW TO

1. You will begin with seated mountain poses again.

2. Now scoot forward. If you are not sure of your balance yet you can stay back. Remember to hold on the sides of your chair for balance. If you feel it is better, you can get a chair with arms for this exercise.

3. Stretch your legs forwards so that they are as straight and level as they can be.

4. Inhale and point your toes forward, then exhale as you pull your toes back. Remember your hands are on your chair for balance or your thighs if you are okay with doing it that way.

5. Repeat the exercise ten times or as many times as you feel comfortable.

6. Now repeat the same series again, this time you will exhale when you point your toes forward and inhale when you pull back your toes.

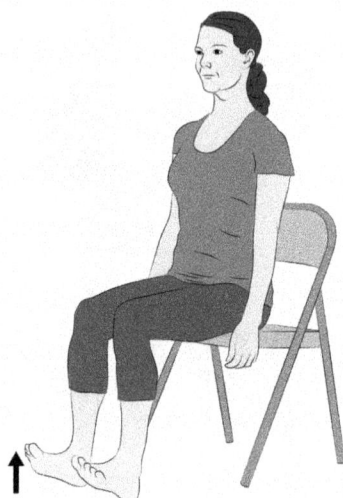

TOE TAPS

DURATION: 2 TO 4 MINUTES

NOTE

Toe taps can help burn more calories and rev up your metabolism. It will work your ankles, shins and feet. It will stimulate your brain and relieve shin splints as well.

HOW TO

1. You will need to sit at the edge of your seat while maintaining your seated mountain pose.

2. Keep your heels on the floor and tap your toes up and down. Keep your posture and focus on your breath.

3. Tap toes on the right foot ten times. Tap the left toes.

4. Tap as fast as you can. Then tap very slowly. Repeat again.

You can try doing it on both feet at the same time.

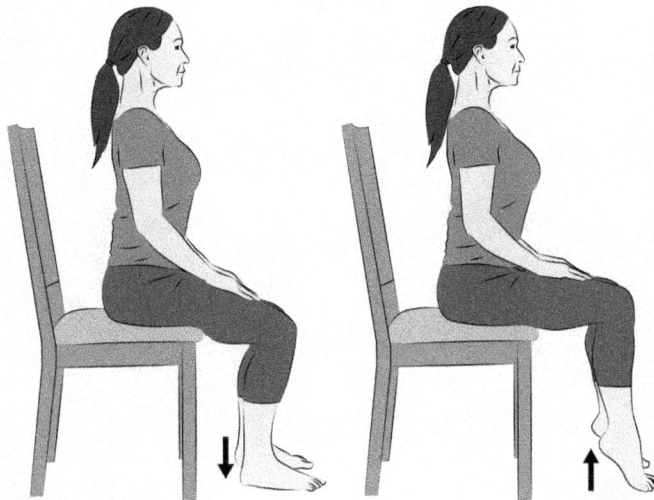

HEEL RAISES

DURATION: 2 TO 4 MINUTES

NOTE

Heel raises will work your inner thighs and calf muscles. They will also help increase your range of motion in the ankle joint.

HOW TO

1. Seat the edge of the chair in your relaxed seated mountain pose. If you can't sit too far out because of injury or back pain, it's fine.

2. Start with your right heel. Lift it ten times. Breathe on the raise and exhale when you put the heel down.

3. Do the same thing with your left heel.

4. Do the sequence with both heels now, at the same time.

5. Now, alternate between left and right for a total of twenty lifts.

6. If you want a challenge, you can increase the speed, doing it faster and faster. This is not mandatory. It is only advised once you have gotten used to the exercise and you want to make it more challenging for yourself.

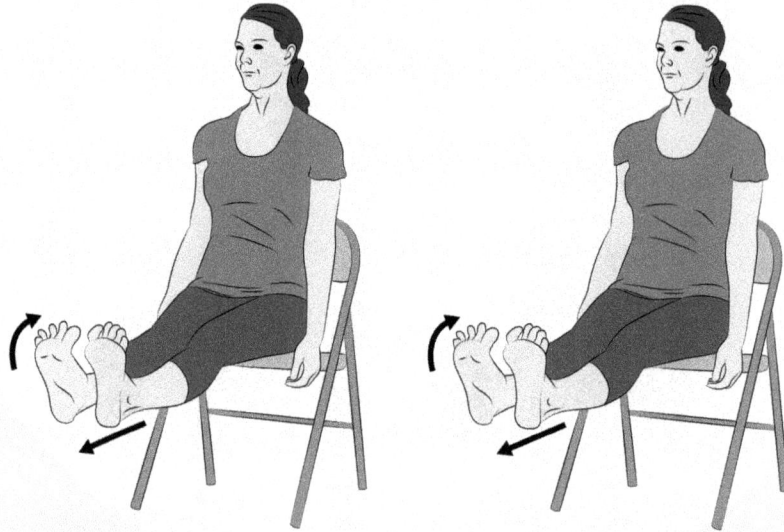

SPREAD AND SQUEEZE

DURATION: 2 TO 4 MINUTES

We are often unaware of how many muscles in our feet go rarely used or stretched. This exercise is very good for preventing common toe issues. It improves overall toe, feet, and ankle health.

HOW TO

1.   Again, we begin with our relaxed seated mountain pose.

2.   Hold on the sides of your chair and lift your legs up as much as you can.

3.   Now squeeze your toes together, as if you are trying to fit them in a small shoe.

4.   Hold this for a few seconds then spread them as wide as you can, like you are trying to use them as a net. It doesn't matter if your toes won't be as wide apart, with experience they will spread more.

5.   However, try to focus on your pinkie toe and attempt separating it from the fourth toe. All that matters is that you are trying, don't get frustrated if it doesn't happen. Focus on doing this on one foot at a time. For a challenge you can try doing both at the same time.

6.   Now spread and squeeze about ten times.

7.   For a challenge increase the number of repetitions and do it faster and cleaner.

8.   Keep your breath steady and regular through the whole exercise for maximum results.

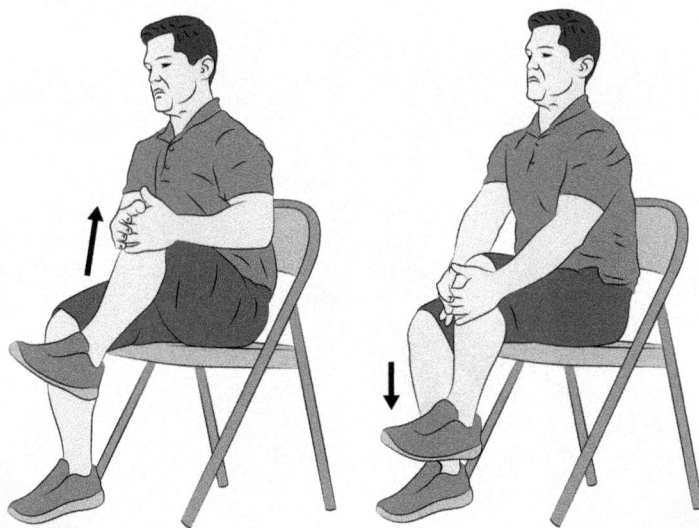

KNEE HUGS

DURATION: 1 TO 4 MINUTES

This exercise helps with stretching your gluteal muscles and lower back, it can help with relieving lower back pain as well.

HOW TO

1. Scoot a little forward in your chair then assume the seated mountain pose.

2. Lace your fingers across the right knee to grab it. Then pull your right knee towards your chest. Pull it as high towards your chest as you can get it. Respect your body if it tells you to stop at a certain level and hold there.

3. Put your leg down and pull it up again. You can repeat this up to ten times. Breathe in as you pull up your leg and breathe out when you put it back down.

4. Repeat with your left leg, not forgetting to link your breathing.

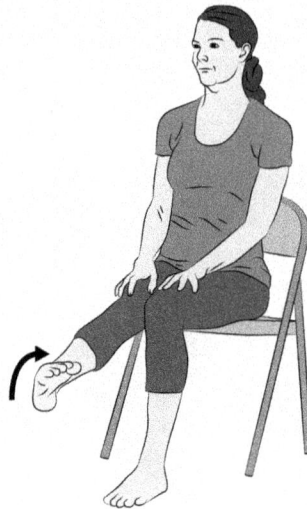

TRACING ALPHABETS

DURATION: 4 TO 10 MIN

NOTE

Tracing the alphabet helps with mobility and flexibility, It will also work many of the muscles in your leg. It is more challenging than many of the other exercises we have done. If you are prone to cramps, this is a good exercise.

HOW TO

1. We begin with the seated mountain pose. Ensure your breathing is steady and you are relaxed throughout the exercise.

2. Lift your dominant foot as high as you can make it and trace the alphabet in the air. There are two ways to do this. You can move your entire leg, which will put muscles up your leg. If you can just move your ankles, that will work your foot and ankles. You can also do both, do the first half by moving your entire leg, and do the second half by moving only your ankle.

3. Then move and do the same with your other leg. With your less dominant leg the exercise will be harder.

4. Experiment with different speeds. If it feels alright and you can breathe in and out at regular intervals, like per two letters traced.

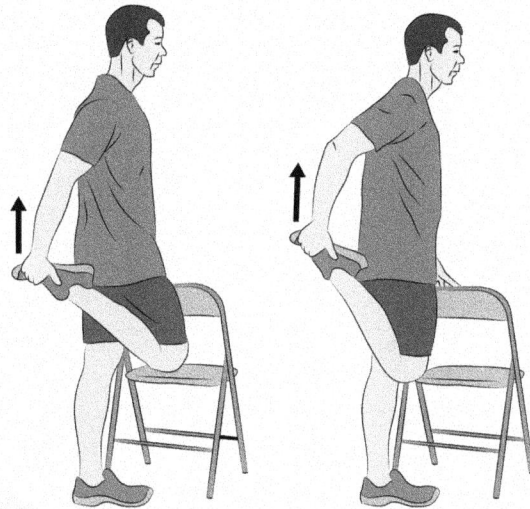

QUAD STRETCHES

DURATION: 1 TO 3 MINUTES

NOTE

Quad stretches are good for the leg muscles, hip flexors and quadriceps. The problem is, often we don't have the balance we need to pull this off, which is where the chair comes in.

HOW TO

1. Stand behind your chair and hold on to it with your dominant hand for balance.

2. Now reach back with your free hand and grab the corresponding foot. Pull it up and draw the foot to your butt. Be gentle.

3. Now hold the position for five to ten breaths.

4. Change sides and do the same thing,

This is a tough exercise especially when you struggle with maintaining balance. Some of you may not even be flexible enough to draw your foot closer to your butt. You can skip this exercise. Or you can do it with the help of a partner, if the grip on the chair is slippery or you are worried about your balance.

NECK AND HEAD EXERCISES

Routines in this section are focused on the head and neck. They are good for relieving tensions and engendering a more relaxed feel. You can do these anyway or even add them to your warm-up routine but they also work as part of a regular yoga routine.

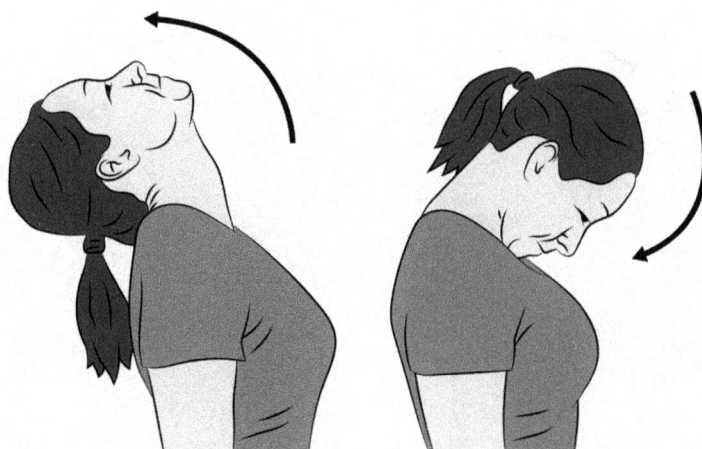

HEAD UP AND DOWN

DURATION: 2 TO 4 MINUTES

NOTE

Perfect for the neck muscles and for relaxation.

HOW TO

1. Assume the seated mountain pose and make sure your feet are hip-width apart.

2. Lift your head up as you inhale, and when you put your head back down you must exhale. Keep your torso still, make sure that movement only occurs in your head and neck.

3. Repeat the exercise fifteen to twenty times.

4. Keep your shoulders down and relaxed during the exercise.

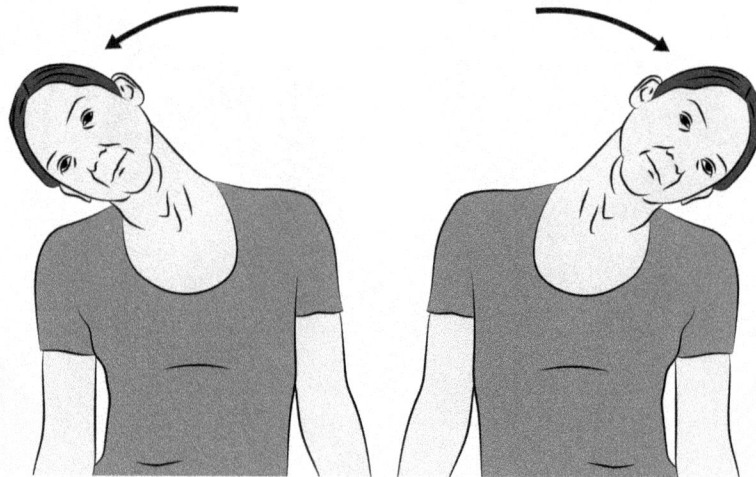

SIDE-TO-SIDES

DURATION: 2 TO 4 MINUTES

NOTE

Great for the neck and the upper chest. It will help loosen up things and help you relax as well.

HOW TO

1. In this exercise all you do is drop your head from side to side. Throughout, ensure you are sitting tall, and your shoulders are relaxed.

2. Inhale, as you drop your left arm towards your left shoulder and then exhale when you return your head back to the center. This means you have to hold the dip for about three seconds at a time or however long you feel comfortable holding your breath. Just keep breathing regularly and not too distressing.

3. Dip your right ear towards your right shoulder and repeat the same routine.

4. Don't repeat one side more than once before switching to another. Repeat the exercise ten to fifteen times and increase the repetitions for more of a challenge. Alternatively to make it more challenging, as you get used to it, you can hold your breath just a bit longer.

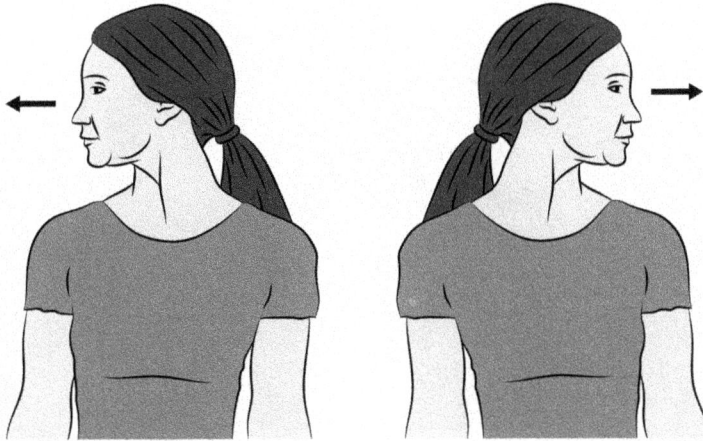

TURNING LEFT AND RIGHT

DURATION: 2 TO 4 MINUTES

This exercise will add more mobility in your head and neck region, and it also works the shoulders a bit.

HOW TO

1. While inhaling, turn your head to the left as far as you can take it. If you encounter too much resistance and pain at a certain point, stop.

2. When you exhale, turn the head as far back left. On inhalation you will return it to the other side and so on.

3. Repeat these ten to twenty times, depending on how it's treating you. You can experiment with moving your head just a little slower to challenge yourself but don't overdo it.

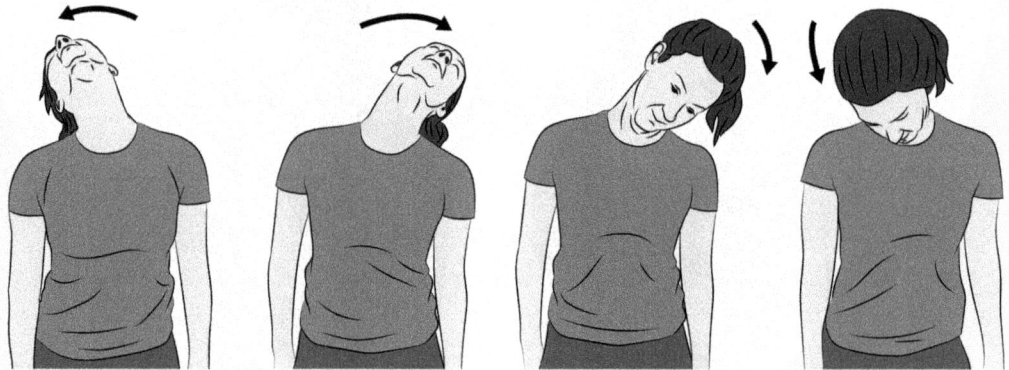

UP AND DOWN WHILE LOOKING

DURATION: 3 TO 4 MINUTES

NOTE

A slight variation on head turns that access more muscles in the neck and the shoulder.

HOW TO

1. While seated in our favorite position. Turn your head to the right. Then on the inhale lift the head up while it is still turned to the side. On the exhale draw the head down while it's still turned.

2. After ten rounds on the right side, get back to center, take a few deep breaths and do the transitions to the left side.

3. Again, you can stop at any point. If it feels too strenuous or painful on your neck., remember our talk on good and bad pain.

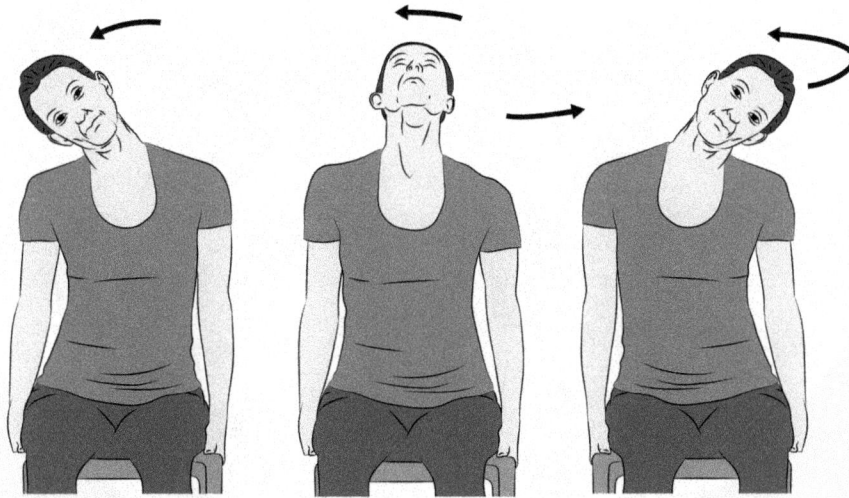

HEAD CIRCLES

DURATION: 2 TO 3 MINUTES

In the warm-up routine we shared in the last chapter you would have done half circles already. As part of your routine, you might incorporate doing full head circles. There are safe ways and harmful ways of doing it.

HOW TO

1. Start with a small movement that is not too wide and slowly build yourself up to a wider movement. This is to prevent injury.

2. Remember to keep your shoulders relaxed and to breathe steadily. You can inhale at the start of each revolution and exhale when one revolution ends.

3. After doing about five rounds, you can make your movement wider. Keep increasing in these similar increments until your chin touches your collarbone or you have reached your full range.

4. If you start counterclockwise repeat the same thing again clockwise, starting small with measured breaths to much wider movements.

5. Sit upright throughout the entire exercise and keep your shoulders down and relaxed.

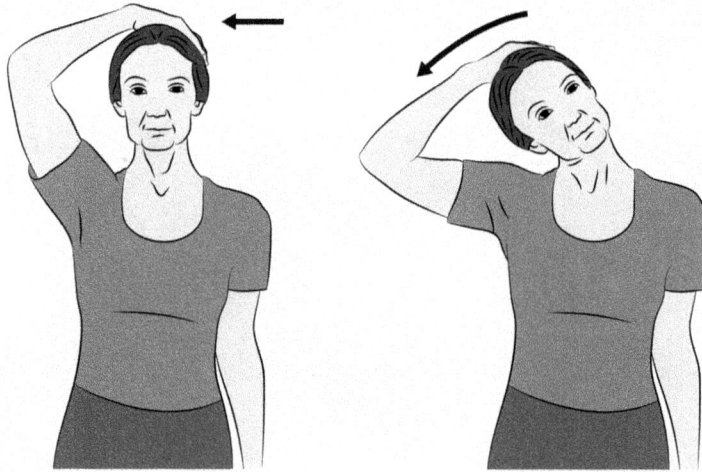

HEAD ASSISTED SIDE STRETCHES

DURATION: 1 TO 3 MINUTES

NOTE

Access the neck and shoulder muscles, relieving tension and helping with relaxation.

HOW TO

1. While you are looking forward, take your right arm over your head to the left side and drop your palm to your left ear. Then drop your head to the right side, towards your shoulder. Pull your ear or gently press your head a little towards your right shoulder. Be gentle, don't force things. Don't use too much pressure; the safest way is to slightly pull your ear too. You should feel a stretch on the left shoulder. Hold the position for 10 deep breaths.

2. To make things interesting, drop your chin toward your right armpit and hold for ten more breaths.

3. Repeat on the other side using your left hand. When you do this exercise, keep the arm that is not on your head relaxed and falling to the side for maximum effect.

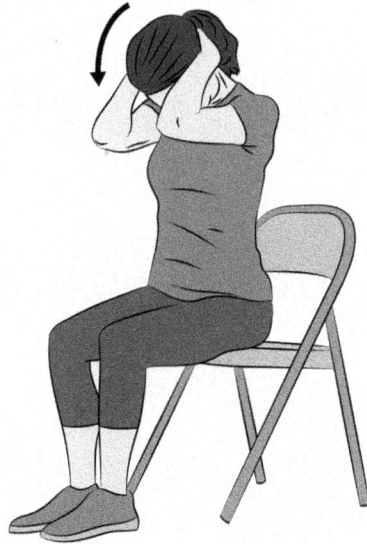

FORWARD BOW

DURATION: 2 TO 4 MINUTES

NOTE

Good for the back, spine, head and neck muscles.

HOW TO

1. Lace your hands behind your head and place your chin on your chest. Now narrow your elbows so that they move closer together. Be careful not to make the distance between them too narrow. Just focus on keeping them pointing straight ahead instead of at each other.

2. When doing this, ensure that you're seated upright. This will help stretch your upper back and spine.

3. Take eight deep breaths. You can make it less if you feel uncomfortable

4. When you are done, lift your head up to a straight position and take 9 more deep breaths. If you feel discomfort, you can drop your head back, so you are looking at the ceiling and deep breaths that way.

SHOULDERS, ARMS AND HANDS

The exercises in this section are targeted at the arms and the shoulders. Aimed at bringing relief and releasing tension. They will also help with mobility and flexibility of the arms.

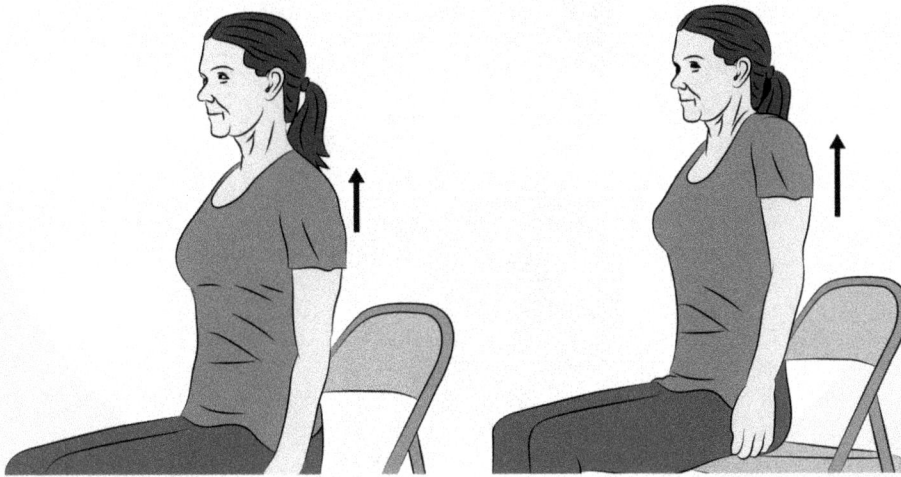

TENSING AND RELAXING SHOULDERS

DURATION: 4 TO 6 MINUTES

NOTE

Builds more awareness of your muscles and helps you relax and relieve tension.

HOW TO

1. While seated upright in the seated mountain pose, scoot toward the edge of the chair.

2. Inhale and lift your shoulder up high towards your ears, in a tensing motion. Hold this for two or three seconds. On exhalation, drop and relax your shoulders.

3. Repeat ten to fifteen times. You can hold for longer, for more of a challenge. Don't forget to link your breathing and avoid rushing this one, as the secret is in those moments of tension and release. You can do this longer if you wish.

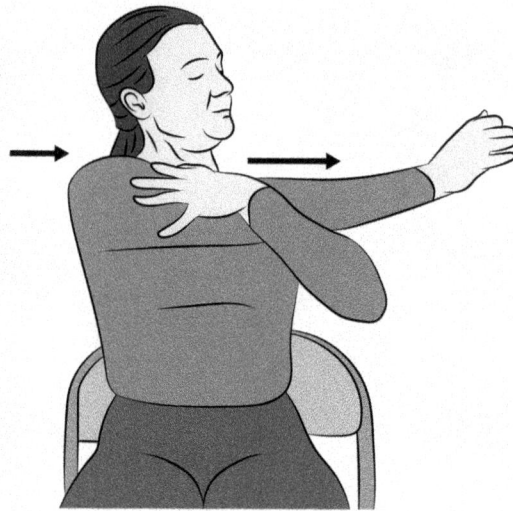

ARM CROSSES

DURATION: 2 TO 5 MINUTES

NOTE

This exercise will help work your outer shoulder, biceps and rear deltoid.

HOW TO

1. Make sure you are on the edge of your chair in the seated mountain pose.

2. Take your right arm across your chest to the other side. Put your left arm over your right elbow or right next to it and press your right arm towards your body. Take seven to ten breaths while holding your right arm in this position. Ensure your shoulders are positioned away from your ears as you do this.

3. Repeat the same procedure on the left side.

4. You can extend the duration as you grow more accustomed to this exercise.

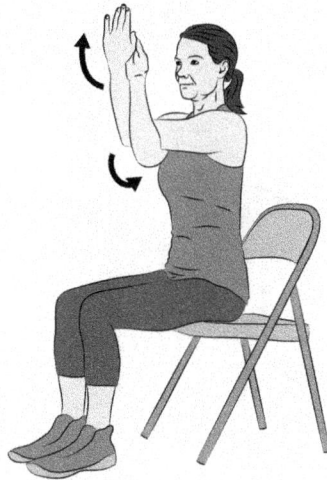

DOUBLE CROSSES

DURATION: 3 TO 5 MINUTES

NOTE

Helps with flexibility and works the arm muscles.

HOW TO

1. This exercise is good for your shoulders, wrists, and arms It will help relieve some pain, tension, and improve flexibility

2. Seated in the mountain pose, raise your arms so that they are about shoulder height high.

3. Now cross your arms by putting one arm under the other. If you can't, just make sure they cross, making an 'X'.

4. Now attempt crossing your arms again towards your wrist and have the palms of each hand press against each other. If you can't have your palms facing each other, you can press the back of your hands together.

5. Hold this pose and take ten deep breaths.

6. Now switch arms and try to do it again. While doing this exercise it is important to lift your elbows a little higher while keeping your shoulder relaxed. You will feel a pull at the back of your shoulder, it's a good sign. To intensify the exercise, you can hold longer breaths prolong the double cross.

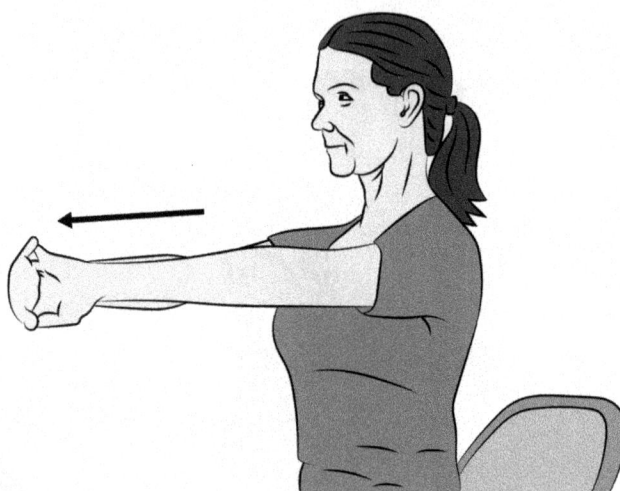

HIGH ALTAR ARMS

DURATION: 2 TO 4 MINUTES

This exercise works tremendously well for the arms, wrists, shoulders and sides.

HOW TO

1. While seated toward the edge of your chair, stretch your arms out in front of you. Then interlace your fingers and turn your palms away from your body. You will feel mild pain on the inside of your wrists, just below the palms when you do that. The harder you press forward the more pain you will exert, so just stretch to the amount that you are comfortable with. You should also feel your triceps, elbows and fingers get worked. This is good as long as you don't overdo it. You should focus on pushing with your wrists and elbows.

2. Take five to ten breaths.

3. While maintaining the stretch, lift your arms slowly above your head, so that you have your knuckles staring down the top of your head. When you move your arms, do so slowly, making sure you are not tensed up in the torso. You feel your shoulder get a little tight, that is fine and remember to gently push up until you encounter some resistance. Don't overdo it.

4. Take five to ten breaths.

5. Focus on pushing with your wrists and elbows when you get into the stretch, not so much with the shoulders.

6. Stop, assume the seated mountain pose. Then repeat the whole exercise for one more round. You can do a couple more rounds for an extra challenge.

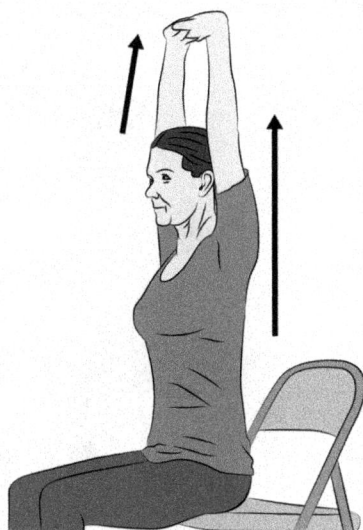

HIGH ALTAR LIFTS

DURATION: 2 TO 5 MINUTES

NOTE

High altar lifts are a variation on the previous exercise.

HOW TO

1. You begin with the high alter pose, with your arms outstretched and palms facing towards the ceiling. Then you lower your hands toward your head, as if you are bringing down a weight that is seated on top of them. This will bring the elbows outward and work your triceps. As you bring down the invisible weight, slightly lean your head forward, and as you touch your head or get close to it, lift up, stretching the arms again in a high altar position.

2. Link deep breaths with the lifting and lowering. You can inhale when you bring down your arms and exhale on the lift.

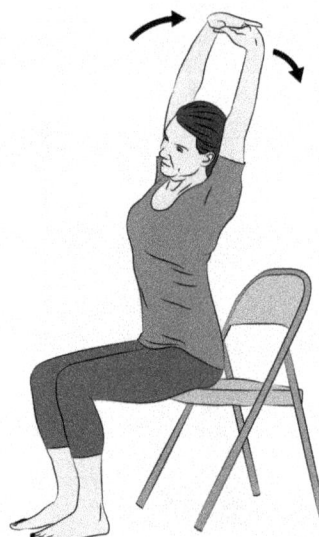

HIGH ALTAR SIDE TO SIDE

DURATION: 2 TO 5 MINUTES

NOTE

Another variation that will help stretch the sides and tone the arms, in addition to the benefits offered by the high alter pose.

HOW TO

1. Begin with the high alter pose (with your interlaced outstretched hands above your head, palms to the ceiling).

2. While maintaining that pose, bend to the right side and hold, while still facing forward (bend to the side). While in this position take five deep breaths, and return to the center

3. Hold the high alter position and take two deep breaths before transitioning to leaning to the left side and holding the pose for five deep breaths.

4. Repeat this exercise at least three times on each side. You can lengthen the time for more of a challenge, but it is advised you start slowly lest you ache too much.

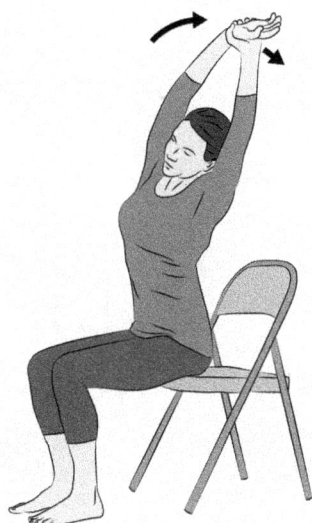

WRIST PULL SIDE LEANS

DURATION: 2 TO 5 MINUTES

1. Raise your hands high, as you did in the high alter pose. Lean to the right side as if you are doing a high altar side to side. Instead of having your fingers interlaced as in the first example, you will use your right hands to grab your wrist. Then pull the left arm by the wrist, further into the right lean. You should feel a tug just beneath your shoulders

2. Take five deep breaths. An alternative to the other side.

3. Do this three times on each side.

If you want the exercise to be more challenging do not pull harder on your arm. You can add more breaths on each lean to prolong the hold.

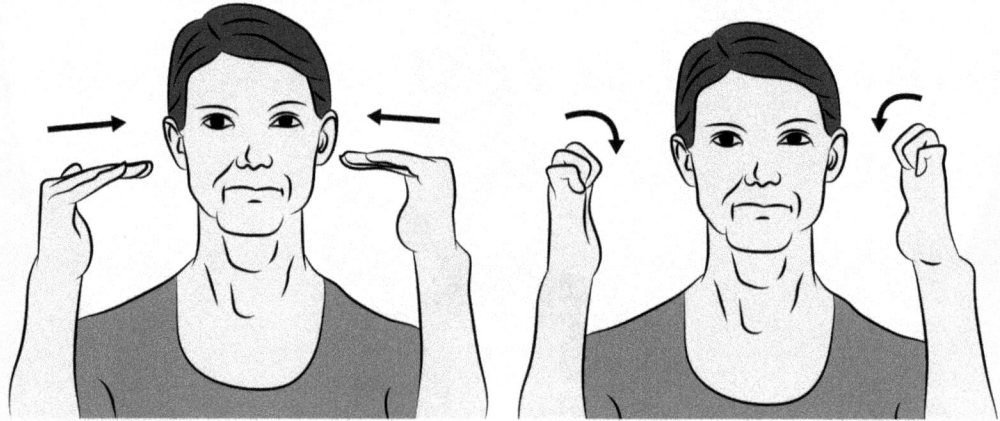

WRIST WORKOUT

DURATION: 2 TO 5 MINUTES

This exercise is good for hand relief, preventing carpal syndrome and similar problems with the hand.

HOW TO

1. Raise your arms with your elbows bent. Raise your elbows to about chest height.

2. Raise your hands straight palms facing each other.

3. Then bend your fingers so that they are facing the floor. You bend the fingers at the knuckles. Your entire hand should make a right angle at this point.

4. Return to the initial straight palm form and then fold the upper part of your fingers so that they look like claws. Try to get your fingertips to touch your palms.

5. Lastly squeeze your fingers into a fist. Keep repeating this for at least twenty times.

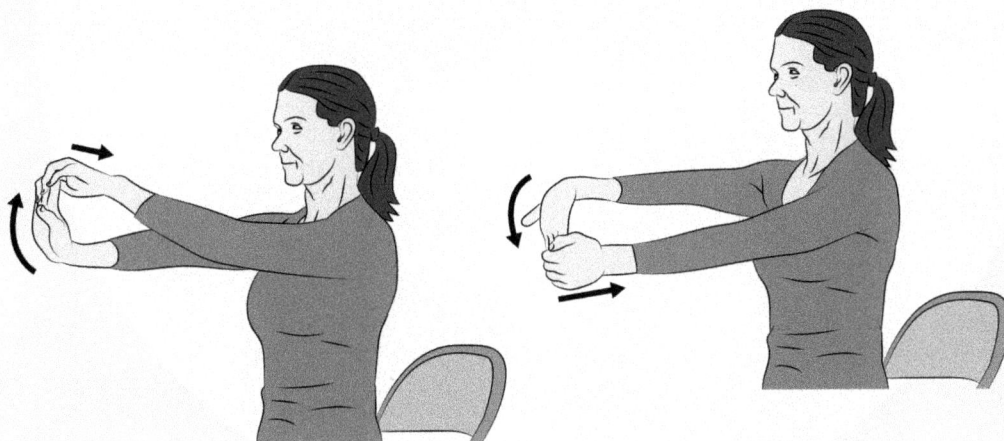

HAND PULLS

DURATION: 2 TO 5 MINUTES

HOW TO

1. While in a seated mountain pose, put your left arm in front of you and make the 'stop' signs gesture with it. Now take your right hand and pull the fingers of your right hand towards your body.

2. Don't pull too hard. Focus on finding a sweet spot and holding the positions for between 30 to 60 seconds.

3. While pulling, remember to take deep breaths.

4. When you are done, switch to the other hand.

5. Repeat another round, this time the 'stop' sign gestures upside down. Be careful with this one as it can get painful if you pull hard without thinking.

I recommend you hold it for at least 30 seconds, but if you find yourself struggling to keep the hand up for that long, it is okay. You can do it until the point you feel is enough. When you are starting, there is no need to rush things. The more you do the exercises, the easier and more tolerable all this will become.

TORSO

In this section, I'm going to look at some exercises that are perfect for the upper body. They're good for building strength, toning and the core.

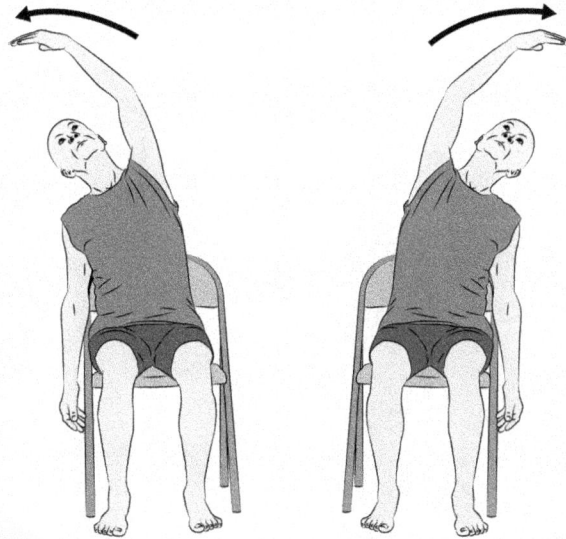

SIDE BEND

DURATION: 2 TO 4 MINUTES

NOTE

We will begin with simple side bends. These are good for abdominal muscles; they can also be good for the hips and help with the flexibility of the spine. We're doing side bends on a chair because trying any of these poses while you are standing up can be very difficult. A chair provides a lot of safety with a lot of the exercises in this section.

HOW TO

1. Beginning in our seated mountain pose, we will sweep both arms from the sides up so that they're pointing towards the ceiling. As we lift our hands, we have to inhale. Then drop your right arm to the side while your left arm is still pointing towards the ceiling.

2. Now bend towards the right side. When you bend, you can keep your right arm straight pointing towards the floor. Or you can grab onto your arm or the chair for balance while you bend to the right side with your left arm reaching to the right side.

3. We don't have to hold this pose for any longer than we want to, so we can just immediately switch to the other side by lifting up our right arm and dropping our left arm. The trick is to inhale when you are transitioning and exhale once you reach the other side with your arm. Each time you reach over towards the other side with your arm, make sure it goes over your head, so that the inside of your elbow gets as close as possible to your head.

4. Keep going from side to side for about 15 times. Remembering to exhale whenever you reach the other side and to inhale during transition.

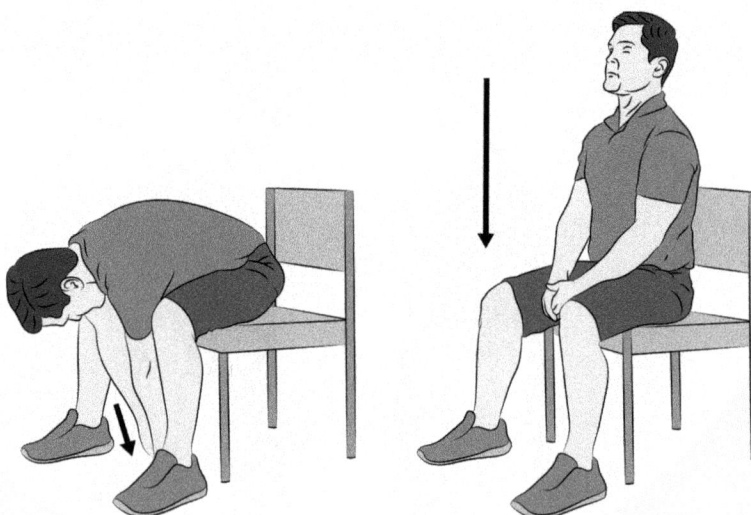

FORWARD FOLD

DURATION: 1 TO 2 MINUTES

NOTE

Forward fold is going to help with stress and high blood pressure

HOW TO

1. Beginning in the seated mountain pose. Inhale deeply and exhale and as you exhale fold forward. That means bring your chest toward your knees in a fold. Before you do this ensure you are seated far back enough in your chair that when you fold forward, you don't risk tipping over forward and falling.

2. A full forward fold won't always be possible. For instance, if you have a big belly you won't be able to reach your knees with your chest. So, all you have to focus on is bending forward as far as your body will allow you. You can wrap your arms behind the knees or hold the back of the chair.

3. Hold this position for about 10 seconds and release. You can hold for a longer time for more challenging exercise.

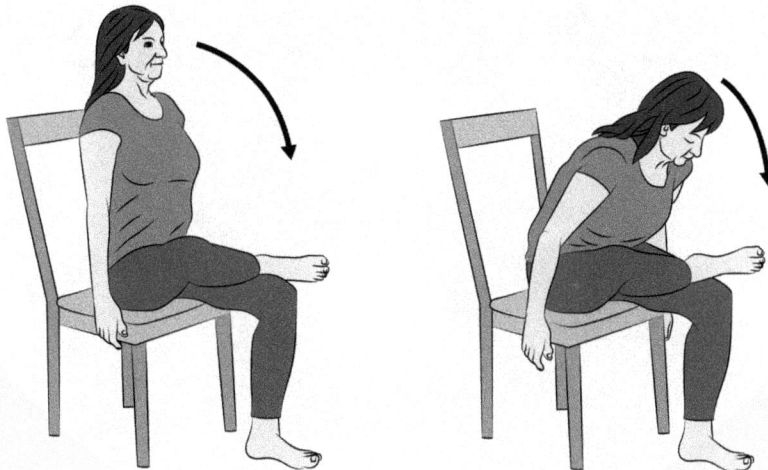

SEATED PIGEON POSE VARIATIONS

DURATION: 2 TO 4 MINUTES

1. While in the seated mountain pose, bring your left ankle over your right ankle. If you want, you can put your left ankle over the right knee.

2. Inhale deeply, then bend forward while your hands are on your knees. Make sure your back is straight, push forward until you are at a 45-degree angle.

3. Do about 10 dips like this while you are exhaling and inhaling.

4. After the dips you can switch sides.

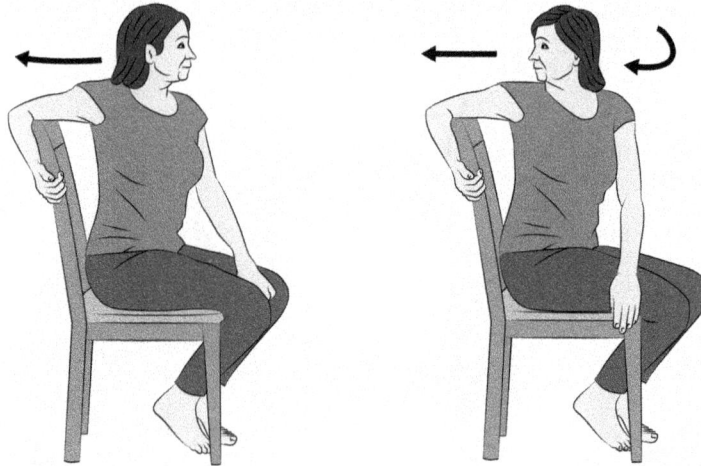

CHAIR TWIST

DURATION: 1 TO 3 MINUTES

Yoga twists help with stretching the back muscles and with spine flexibility. They can also help in lengthening the spine and improving digestion.

1. Place your right hand on the left knee. Place your left arm on top of the backrest. Let the armrest in such a way that your left elbow is pointing right behind you.

2. Hold this position for about 5 to 10 deep breaths and then switch by placing a left hand on the right knee and the right hand on top of the chair's back.

3. Remember to sit tall and straight for the maximum effect. Repeat the sequence at least two times on each side.

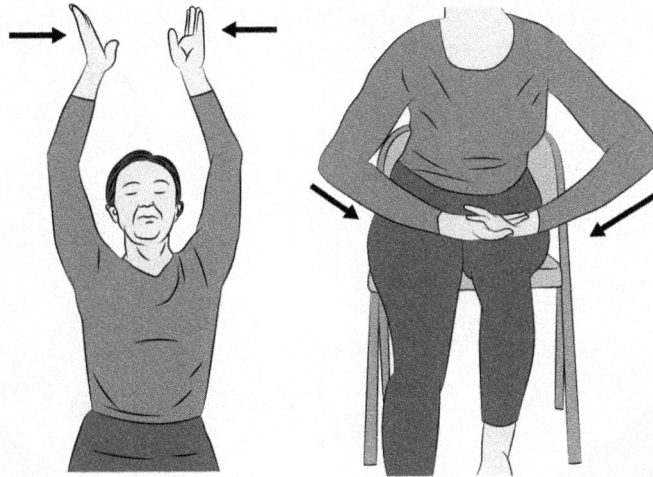

FORWARD FOLD VARIATION

DURATION: 2 TO 4 MINUTES

HOW TO

1. We start by sweeping up arms above our ahead as we inhale. Now stretch your right leg forward so that it sits on its heel on the floor.

2. Now fold forward putting both your hands on your left knee, as if to press down. You don't have to apply a lot of pressure. Afterwards, move your hands to the outstretched right leg from the thighs and trace them down over the knee, shins and down towards your ankle. If you can't reach your ankle on the outstretched leg that is fine just reach as far as you can.

3. Hold this for five to ten seconds. Don't forget to take those deep breaths.

4. Return to the seated mountain pose again. Start the whole sequence over and this time stretch the left leg.

5. You can repeat this two more times before stopping.

For safety and balance ensure you are seated far back enough in your chair.

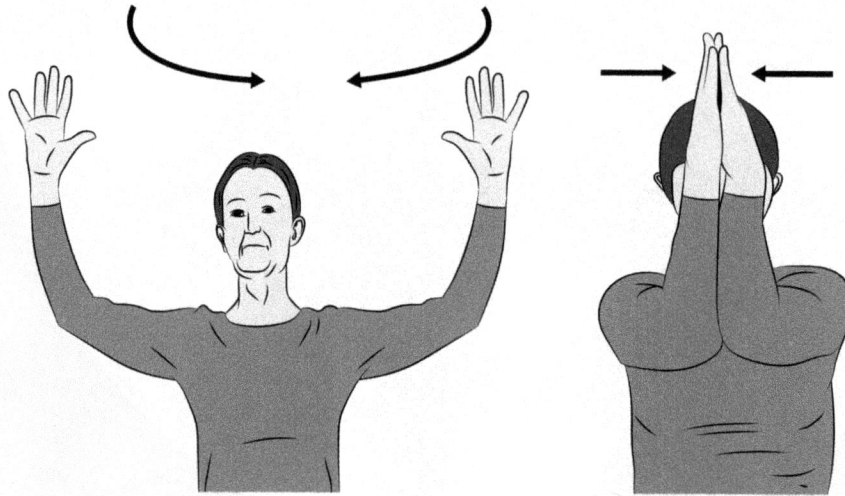

CACTUS FLOWER

DURATION: 2 TO 4 MINUTES

1. While in the seated mountain pose, raise your arms to the side so that your elbows are level with your shoulder. Ensure that they are bent at a 90 degree angle and you are open and facing forwards. Your arms should be on the sides in the same line as your head.

2. While holding this pose, breathe in and pull your arms back behind your. You should feel it in the shoulder blades. This opens up the chest and allows you to take deeper breaths.

3. On the exhale, draw your arms together in front of you so that palms and elbows touch.

4. Repeat this five to ten times, remembering to link your breathing with closing the cactus(drawing arms in front) and opening the cactus(pulling them back).

In another variation of the cactus flower, you can add an additional step after you do the initial exercise. You open the cactus one more time and pull slightly back. Instead of closing the cactus, you instead lift your arms straight on the exhale, straightening the elbows. You repeat this about five to ten times. Alternatively, you can do cactus side bends. You hold the cactus open, and then you do a side bend, hold for a couple of sections, and repeat on both sides five times.

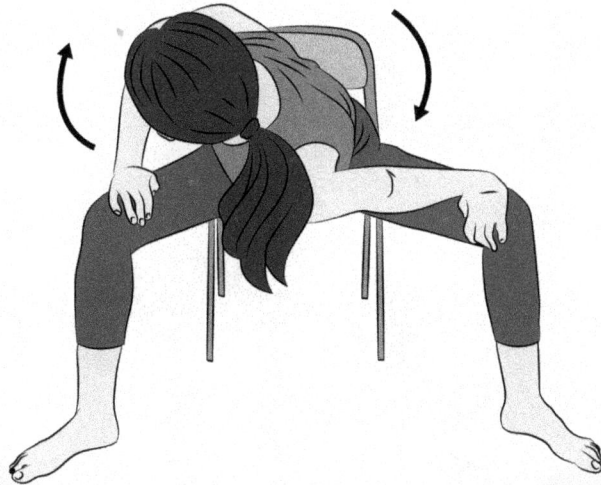

SEATED GODDESS POSE

DURATION: 2 TO 4 MINUTES

1. To get into the seated goddess pose all you have to do is open up your legs as wide as you can get them from the seated mountain pose. Your toes should be pointing out to the sides. Pretend that you are trying to get your legs abreast the front let's of your chair. Open up as much as your body will allow you but not so much you lose balance. You are going to have to lean forward, so it needs to be sturdy.

2. Now take your hands and place them on your knees. Inhale deeply.

3. On the exhale, lean forward(not too much), twist the right shoulder forward and the body to the left side. Turn your head that way too. Your right arm should get straighter while your left arm bends.

4. Comeback to the center. Inhale and the switch sides.

5. Repeat the sequences five to ten times depending on what is most comfortable to you.

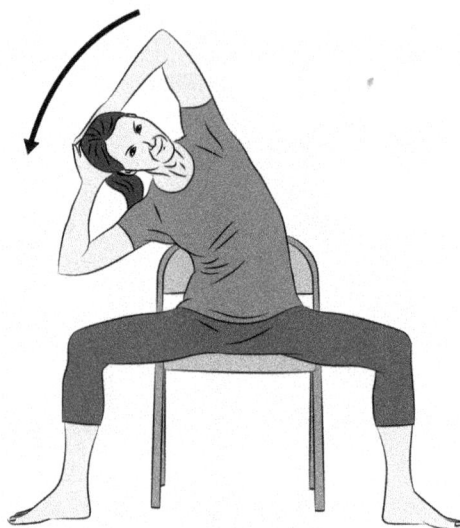

SEATED GODDESS SIDE CRUNCHES

DURATION: 3 TO 6 MINUTES

NOTE

Will work your abs and inner thighs.

HOW TO

1. Assume the seated goddess pose, legs wide apart and feet pointing to the sides. Make sure your balance is still retained.

2. Instead of putting your hands on your knees, lace your fingers together behind your head.

3. Inhale and then side bend towards your right leg. As you do this keep your face looking forwards and your torso looking forward, In other words, don't turn or twist; do a side bend.

4. When you exhale, switch over to the left side.

5. Keep bending side to side, exhaling and inhaling as you do. You can repeat these ten or more times. Pace does not matter as much; the same work is done whether you are doing it slow or fast. Remember to squeeze your waist every time you bend from side to side.

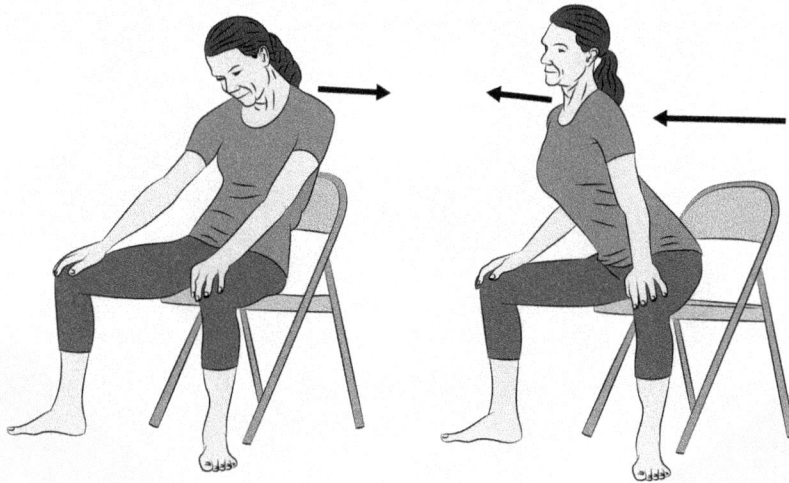

SEATED GODDESS CIRCLES

DURATION: 2 TO 5 MINUTES

These are good for the lower back, abs, and pelvic floor muscles. It also puts some work on your legs too.

HOW TO

1. Sit at the edge of your chair and widen your legs so that your feet are pointing to the sides. Make sure you are seated tall. This is the goddess pose we did earlier.

2. Place your hands on your knees

3. Now, using your abdomen, start circling your torso clockwise, going back into your chair and coming all the way to the front. That means your legs should be firm enough to support your weight when you lean forward in the circling motion. Engage the core and keep going.

4. Take inhale and exhale per circle or half a circle.

5. Now stop at the center after five to ten circles and circle counterclockwise repeating the same sequence.

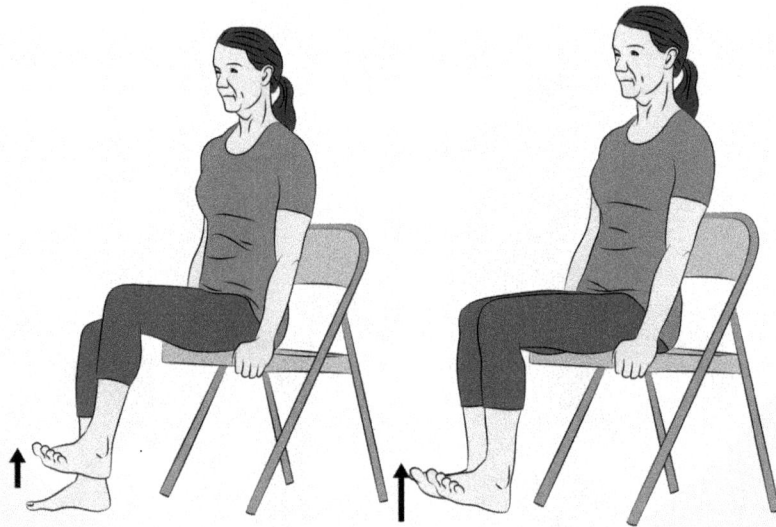

LEG LIFTS

DURATION: 3 TO 5 MINUTES

NOTE

Leg lifts won't just work on your legs, but they are good at stretching the abdomen.

HOW TO

1. Sit towards the edge of your seat. Draw your lower abdomen in and up.

2. Using the energy in your abdominal muscles to lift you up by a few degrees and then hold that position for three to five seconds. Make sure the left is still bent at a 90-degree angle when you raise it. It's better, just imagine you are trying to get your knee just below the height of your belly button.

3. When you do this, ensure you are breathing calming breaths.

4. Switch legs and repeat this for 12 to 15 times. If you can't do that many, it's okay, just do as many as you can handle. Just remember to leverage your core to lift your legs and avoid relying too much on your arms.

5. To make things more challenging you can try to raise both your legs at the same time and hold for the duration of three seconds and then rest. You can repeat this as many times as it works for you. Remember not to raise your feet too high, raising them a little above the pelvis is fine.

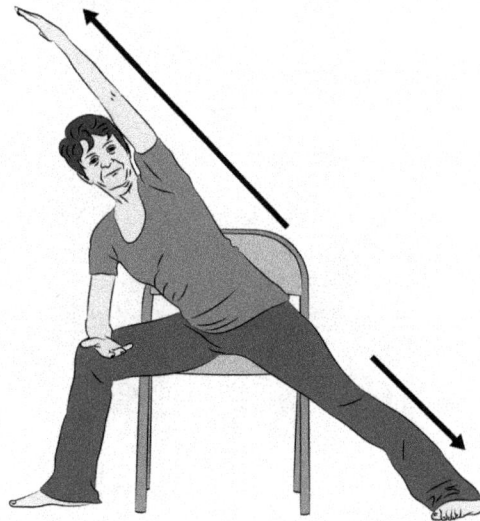

EXTENDED SIDE ANGLE

DURATION: 2 TO 6 MINUTES

NOTE

This exercise is great for the hips, legs and lower back.

HOW TO

1. Scoot over toward the edge of the chair, but firmly seated. Extend your legs to the goddess pose. Then, making sure your left thigh and pelvic area rests on the chair, extend your right leg out to the side into a straight stretch while your left leg stays firm at a 90-degree angle.

2. Rest your left elbow on your left knee.

3. Reach with your right hand to the left side in a side bend. If you can, look up at your hand. Your arm should go over your right ear and overhead.

4. Hold this position and feel all the work your body is doing while you take deep calming breaths.

5. Then switch sides and repeat.

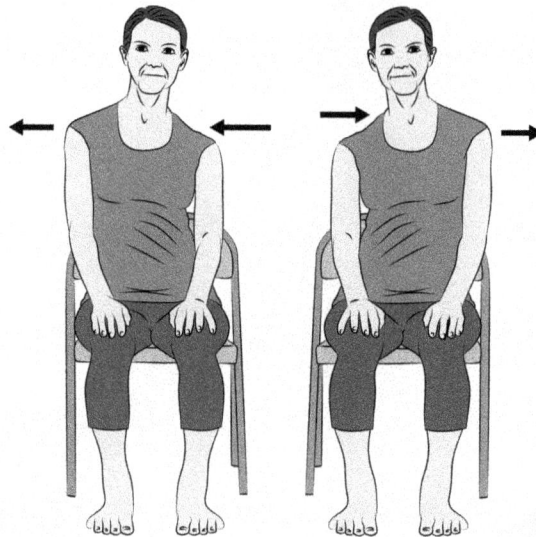

SHIFT SIDES TO SIDES

DURATION: 3 TO 5 MINUTES

1. Sit tall with your feet hip-width apart. Make sure your ankles are right under your knees and your back is straight.

2. Keeping this posture, slide your rib cage left and inhale. When you exhale, slide it to the right side. Ensure it is just your torso moving, that you don't move with your butt or feet.

3. Repeat this movement for up to 20 times. If you can't get as much done, it is okay. It will feel awkward the first time you do this. That is perfectly fine. Just remember to keep your core engaged.

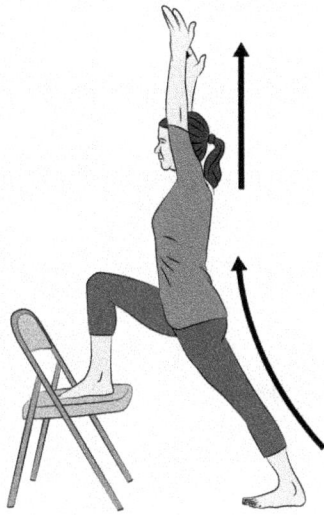

LUNGE

DURATION: 3 TO 5 MINUTES

Perfect for pain in the lower back and stretching the legs. Lunges also work the quadriceps, calves and muscles.

HOW TO

1. Stand in front of your chair and put your right foot on the seat. The chair has to be sturdy and have a back, so an accident does not happen.

2. Now hold the back of the chair and stretch the left leg on your floor. To stretch the left leg on the floor, don't push the back too hard. Just reach for the back of the chair and just let your body do the work.

3. Press the foot on the floor firmly. To avoid injuries don't let the knee pass the ankle too much.

4. Now, hands off the chair and lift both your arms straight up to point at the ceiling. You should feel your body stretch more as you do this.

5. Hold the position for five to ten breaths and then repeat on the left side.

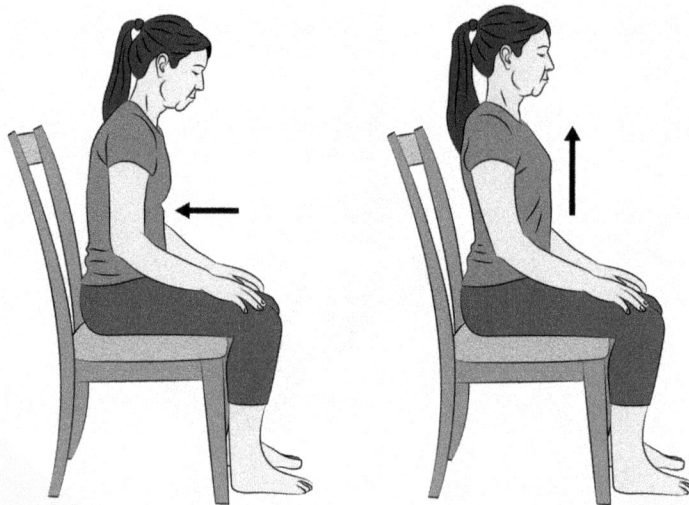

LOWER BACK CIRCLES

DURATION: 2 TO 3 MINUTES

NOTE

This is perfect exercise for the lower back and abdominals.

HOW TO

1. While seated with your hands resting your knees, imagine you will be using your lower half to stir. Instead of rounding your back forward and back backward, you will be concentrating on keeping your thighs relatively straight and using your lower half of your upper body to do circles.

2. Inhale and circle around clockwise.

3. Do this for between six to ten circles and then change direction.

4. Remember to inhale and exhale with each circle or half a circle. You can do this longer if it feels really good.

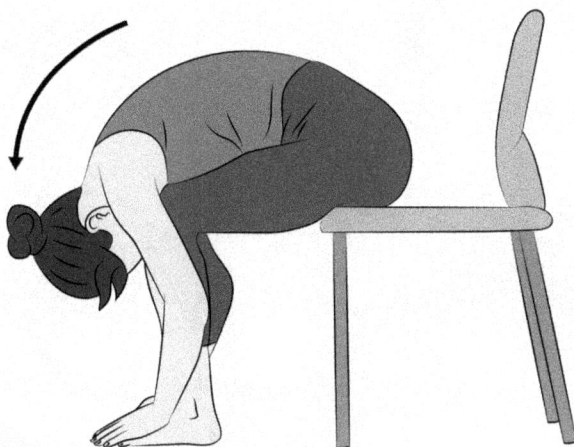

ROLL DOWNS

DURATION: 2 TO 4 MINUTES

These are a great way to open up the vertebrate. They are also good for the back, spine and abdominals.

HOW TO

1. Begin with the seated mountain pose, instead of having your hands on your knees let them hang to the sides.

2. From your head downwards, start to slowly round down through the spine. Exhalation will help with the descendent. Keep going down slowly, following your back until your head. Pretend you are letting your head fall forward without trying to use your torso to hold it. Instead let your vertebrae roll down starting right beneath the back of the head.

3. On inhalation, slowly unroll the vertebrae again to sit up straight and tall. Ensure you draw your belly button to help your back as you round up.

4. Repeat these five to ten times, rounding down and rounding up.

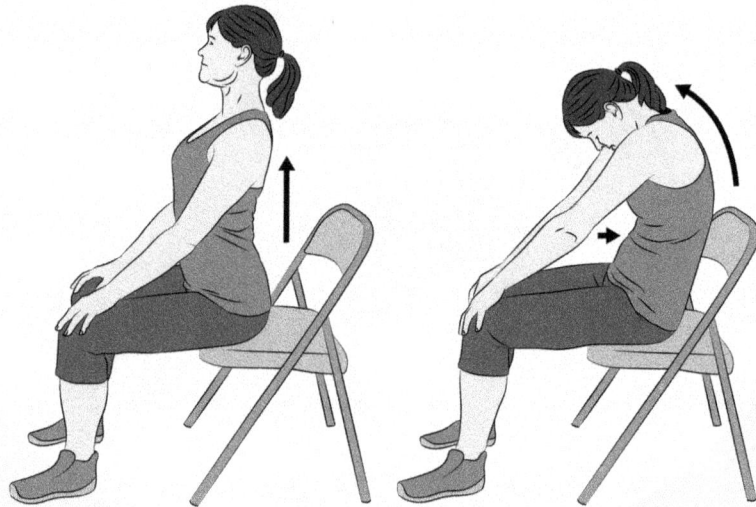

CAT AND COW

DURATION: 1 TO 3 MINUTES

NOTE

You will be familiar with the cat and cow pose, it is one of the exercises we worked on in our warm-up chapter. It's one of the most basic exercises in all of chair yoga and it happens to be very good for your back and abdominals.

HOW TO

1. While sitting in the seated mountain pose with your hands on your knees and feet flat on the floor, inhale. As you inhale, point your chest up, as if towards the sky, leaving your lower back and hips behind. Your back will be arched.

2. Look up, squeeze your shoulders together, while holding the pose. This is the cow pose.

3. As you exhale, deflate the chest and allow your midsection to fall in and go as deep as the tailbone. Your back should rise, as if that of a cat.

4. Repeat ten times at least.

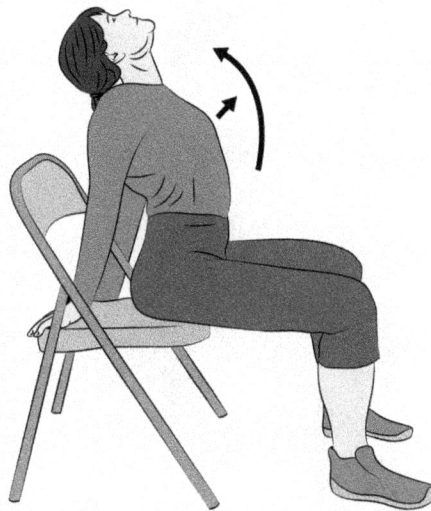

BACKEND ARCH

DURATION: 1 TO 3 MINUTES

NOTE

The exercise is good at working your lower and upper back. It's very good at stabilizing the core and increasing flexibility.

HOW TO

1. Sit at the edge of your chair. Then place your hands behind you on the seat of the chair, pointing towards the chair's back legs away from the hips.

2. Use your fingertips to prop yourself up. Then arch forward, drawing your back in and upwards to lift your lower back. Arch all the way up until you feel it all the way up you back towards your shoulder blades.

3. Hold this position and take five to ten deep breaths. You get to repeat this multiple times if you want more of a challenge.

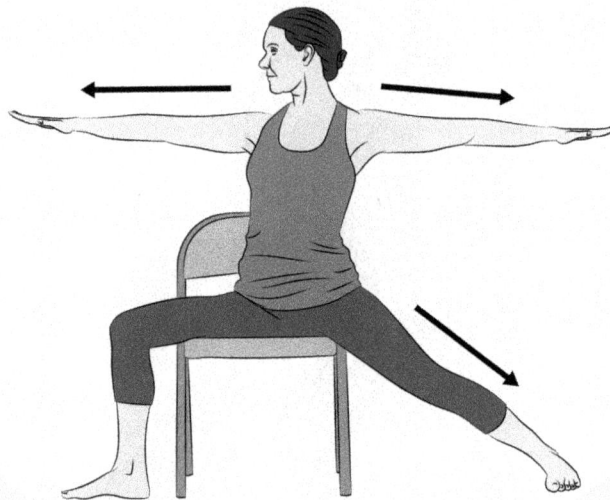

WARRIOR POSE

DURATION: 1 TO 3 MINUTES

NOTE

It works on your buttocks, hips, abs, arms and legs. It is great for building balance and strength.

HOW TO

1. Now sit to the side of your chair, so instead of your back facing the back of the chair it is facing the other side. Seats so at that least your butt is at the edge of the other side of the seat.

2. If you are looking towards the right side, take your outer leg, which will be your left off the chair and stretch back behind you. You should ensure that your right leg is firmly planted on the floor at a right angle, as your left leg stretches out behind you and with your thigh, leg and pelvic area on the seat of the chair.

3. Now, extend your arms to the side, and hold them out like you would the wings of an airplane, twist your torso so that it faces where the chair is facing.

4. Hold this position for five to ten breaths.

5. Afterwards, go back to your starting position and repeat the exercise on the side. You can repeat this sequence a couple of times if you want.

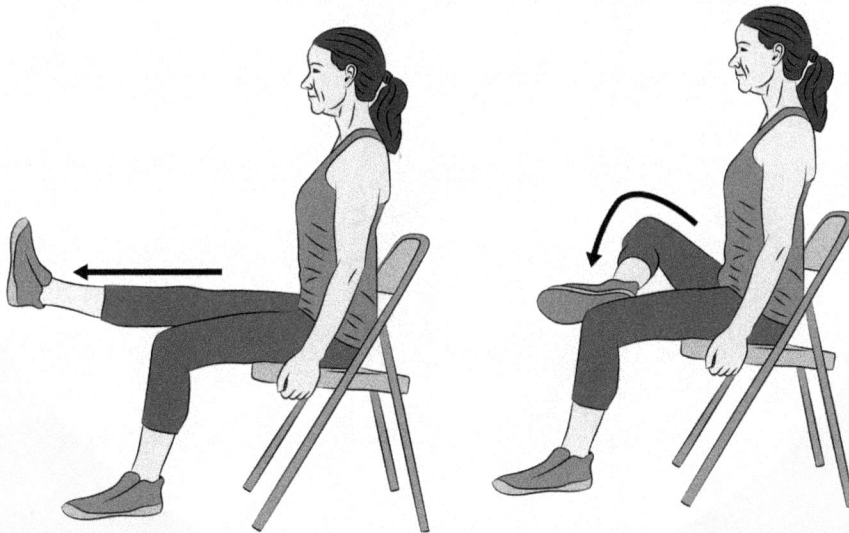

MARCHING FLOW

DURATION: 3 TO 6 MINUTES

NOTE

This is a great exercise for the external rotators, quads, inner thighs and the core. It also strengthens the legs and really awakens your muscles.

HOW TO

1. Sit comfortably in the chair with your feet hip-width apart. Make sure you are seated tall.

2. Inhale and straighten one of your legs in front of you, up in the air, so that they are level or raise above the seat of your chair. Seating comfortably in the middle of the chair instead of the edge will make this easier. If you can't raise your leg that high, it is fine, you will get better at it, no need to rush. Use your core for strength and be careful not to lose your tall posture.

3. When you exhale, bend the knee of your extended foot and put it's ankle on top of the knee of the planted leg. You may need to use your hands to lift your leg. But if you are struggling there is no need to get your ankle up there. You can just have your calf touch the sheen of your planted foot and then put it down.

4. On the next inhale, switch legs and repeat the sequence. Repeat the whole thing eight to ten times.

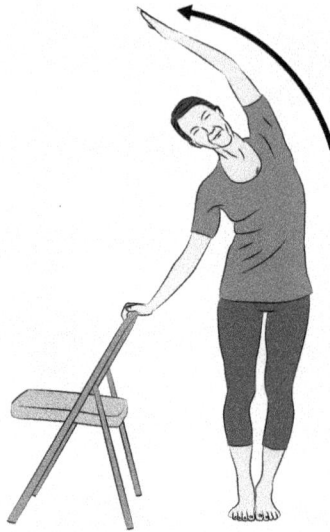

STANDING SIDE STRETCH

DURATION: 1 TO 3 MINUTES

HOW TO

1. Stand behind the chair with your right side to the chair. Now, place your right hand on the back of the chair.

2. Inhale and lift your left arm up and over your head in an arching side stretch, like you are leaning against the chair with your side. Hold the position for five to ten breaths. Your shoulder should be down when you do this. You can look up to also stretch your arm.

3. Now, switch sides and do the same thing again. You can repeat this a couple more times.

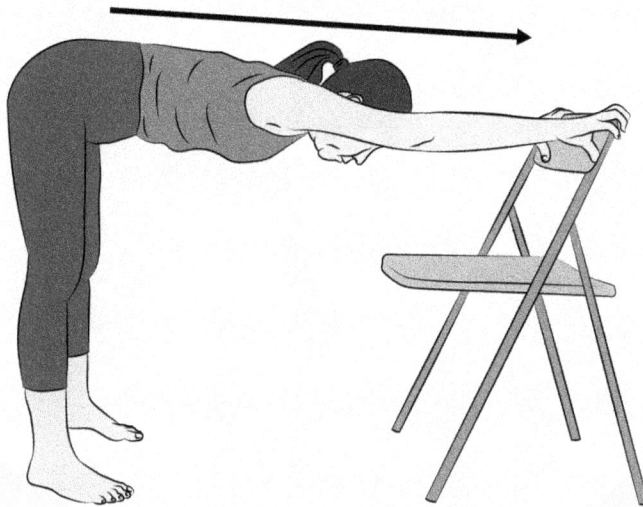

DOWNWARD FACING DOG

DURATION: 1 TO 4 MINUTES

NOTE

Downward facing dog is great for stretching the body. It works great for the arms, back, legs and abs.

HOW TO

1. Stand behind the chair and place your hands on top of the chair back. Ensure your hands are shoulder-width apart.

2. Then walk back until your chest is facing the floor. Hold the positions and engage the stomach, lifting your ribs away from the floor in an arcing motion.

3. You can bend your knees to help straighten yourself more. Hold the position and take five to ten breaths.

4. In another variation you can do the whole exercise by placing your hands on the seat of the chair instead of the back.

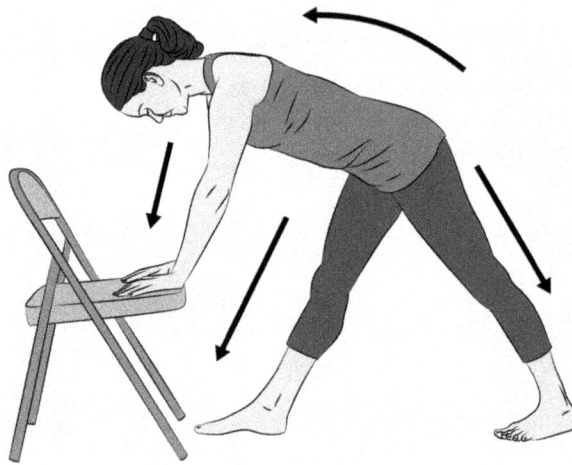

SIDE STRETCH

DURATION: 1 TO 4 MINUTES

NOTE

This helps with keeping hamstrings flexible and it will work your quadriceps, abs and back.

HOW TO

1. Stand facing the chair and put your right foot forward, so your toes are just under the seat of your chair on the floor. Then take your left foot and move it behind you about the same distance as your right left.

2. Now, put the palms of your hands on the edge of the seat, hinging forward with your waist. Don't move your feet, make sure they are securely planted on the floor. Ensure that your back is also straight and flex your quadriceps and muscles above the knees.

3. Take five to ten deep breaths. For a challenge, you can move your chest towards your thigh, but you don't have the exercise as it works fine. Alternate sides and repeat again. You can do this twice or more times. Just don't overdo it. If the pull on your hamstring is uncomfortable, try reducing the stretch by putting your foot close together.

KEY
TAKEAWAY

Many of the routines we will share in upcoming chapters will incorporate these exercises. However, the beauty of the exercises is how they can be done anywhere, whenever you get the chance. I made them easily accessible and versatile because I want them to be easy for the aging population or those with mobility issues. You can reap the benefits without going out of your way to be active.

For instance, as you sit down for breakfast, you can squeeze in a few exercises. You can do the same when using public transport. In the next chapter I will share some routines you can do everyday or whenever you have the space for much longer sessions.

I find that doing these exercises in between activities can really increase your energy levels and keep you fresh and engaged. The beauty of yoga is that it can give you that without being strenuous and intrusive.

Chapter 4
ROUTINES

Exercises are great, but knowing how to combine them into one powerful workout that targets multiple areas of the body, is desirable for many people. The beauty of a yoga routine is how active, meditative, and refreshing it can be. Many people would prefer the transcendental and transformative power of a yoga session over isolated yoga exercises sprinkled throughout the day. This chapter contains routines targeted at building balance, strength, posture, and flexibility

CHAIR YOGA ROUTINE FOR BALANCE

DURATION: 10 TO 15 MINUTES

You will begin seated tall in your chair. You will take deep breaths through the nose, or nose inhaling and mouth exhale (which feels comfortable). You will then bring your right foot forward and start doing foot circles. You can circle the foot five times before circling in the other direction. Once that is done, you will lift your right foot and start doing point and flex. You will bring the point forward with the foot as if using your big toe to point at things and then bring the toes back as if pointing towards yourself. Do this five times. Then switch the sides to repeat the sequence on the left foot. Through this step don't hunch over, keep the tall, seated posture and use your abdomen for strength if necessary.

Afterwards lace your fingers just below your right knee and bring up the knee towards your chest (knee hugs). Repeat this five times and then switch over to the left side. Remember to link your breathing as you do the exercise. The drawing of the knee to your chest should be done when you inhale and when you put it back exhale.

Try to use your abdomen for strength and try to maintain an upright posture. There is an interesting variation you can do on leg hugs. While your leg is drawn to your chest you can cricket your foot two times in both directions. If you don't have the stamina yet to do that, don't worry and just stick with the instructions as is.

If you can, after the leg hug, bring your ankle on top of the other leg's knee and let it sit. You can grab it with your hands and help circle the foot. If you can't put the ankle on top of the foot on the floor is fine. Do this on both sides.

Now, transition into side twists. While seated looking forward, put your left hand on your right knee and grab the back of your seat with your arm and twist to the side. Hold the position for at least five deep breaths and switch over to the other side. If you're keen for a challenge, you can cross your legs and attempt the twist.

Now, go back to your starting position, seated upright and facing forward. Take your arms to the side and loosely shake them up, like there is film on the arms that you want to get rid of. Do this momentarily and then try the same thing with the legs. If you can do the legs and the arms at the same time, it will require more balance and a sturdy chair. Alternatively, you can tap your legs rapidly on the floor.

Revert to your starting position with your hands on your knees and take a few deep breaths.

Then, stand next to your chair. If you are standing on the left side of the chair, put your right hand on the back of the chair for balance. With the front of the foot and toes lightly touching the floor, circle the foot using the legs as if to stir a pot. Do this in both directions. Stop, take a few deep breaths, move to the other side of the chair, and repeat the same sequence. You might feel wobbly as you do this, so ensure that you are holding tight to the back of the chair, and the chair is sturdy. Your foot doesn't have to be loose as you do this but, circling the entire leg with the foot is important. Close your eyes and take deep breaths. Paying attention to your balance after you are done with each side of the chair.

Standing on the side of the chair, lift the leg closest to the chair and outstretch it in front of you. Now do a point and flex exercise on the foot. Begin by pointing the foot forward and then gently putting the back towards yourself and the heel pushes forward. Repeat this at least five times before moving to the other side of the chair and doing the same on the other leg. Don't forget to link your breathing with your movements.

Move to the back of your chair and place your hands on the back of the chair for balance. Now lift up the heels and put them gently down. Do these five to ten times. If there is too much strain, and you are worried about your balance, you can do this one leg at a time. If you are feeling a lot more confident, you can place your hands on your waist and lift up both your heels at the same time. Remember, the more you do this, the easier it will be to do the more advanced exercises, so there is no need to rush if there is something you cannot do yet.

There is a variation to heel lifts where you don't constantly lift them and put them back down gently. In that variation you just lift the heels and hold the position for five to ten breaths. Remember to keep your hands on the chair and not to distribute too much wait to your toes (that might mean not lifting your heels too high).

When your foot comes to the floor you can do some stationary walking. Don't lift your knees too high and be gentle. Do this for ten seconds at least. You can then return to your chair, close your eyes and do some warm-down exercises to conclude the routine, or you may simply close your eyes and do some breathing exercises.

Feel free to incorporate any of the exercises from the last chapter in this routine if you like.

CHAIR YOGA FOR STRENGTH AND FLEXIBILITY

DURATION: 15 TO 20 MINUTES

For this exercise you will be seated the entire time and you will need a small dumbbell or something with comparable weight. You can use a water bottle or a can of vegetables, anything you can get a good grip on. Begin seated tall, fit hip width wide and your ankles right under your knees at a 90-degree angle.

We will begin with shoulder rolls. So, you will roll your shoulders forward for five times or more and then do the same in the opposite direction.

Then inhale, and as you do sweep the arms up to the sides. Right on top of your head put your palms together and then with an exhale, bring your hands down in a prayer hands gesture. You can repeat the sequence three of our times before moving on.

Now, put your hands to the side with the palms facing towards you. And in a straight forward arching motion, lift the arms up until they are pointing up towards the ceiling. Inhale when you lift the arms

up and exhale when you put them down to the sides again. Repeat the sequence three to five times. Remember to use your core as strength if you need it and sit tall.

Lift your arms up one time and hold up pointing at the ceiling. As they are in those positions, you are going to do a forward fold, hinge at the hip and fold forwards with your chest towards your knee. If you can't reach your knees, it's completely fine. All you have to do is fold as far forward as you can, remember to keep your back straight just while you are seated. When you reach the end of your fold you can let the arms down, sit up again and repeat the whole sequence again. Do these three to five times.

Revert back to our beginning seated position and then do heel raises while sitting in this position. When you do heel raises this time, squeeze the calf muscles and gently release them when you put your heels back to the floor. Link the raises with inhalation and the drops with exhalation. The more you raise them up, try to use more and more muscles up your leg for the raises, all the way to the butt. Do this five times.

Return to the starting position with our hands on our knees and I want you to use heel and toe movements to open our legs wide as if we are about to sit in the seated goddess pose. To do this, move both your heels to the outside. After putting them down, move your toes to the outside, repeat this until your legs have opened wide. Then use the same heel toe movements to reverse and get back to our starting position. Inhale when you expand and exhale when you contract. Repeat this three to five times.

Then sit at the edge of the chair and put your feet wide apart but not too wide. Then drop your right knee towards your left calf. Your butt should shift in the chair as you do this, that is fine. Drop your knee so that it points towards the left calf. It shouldn't touch the floor. Hold the seat of the chair behind you for balance. Bring the leg to its original wide position and do the drop with the left knee. Repeat these eight to ten times. Make sure you're relaxed and the movements are smooth.

Then return to the original seating position with your legs parallel and hip-width. Then bring your arms to the side with palms facing forward and raise them up to the side forming a V shape. Now, bend at the elbow forming cactus pose and bring the elbows down towards the sides. You inhale when you bring the arms up and exhale when you bring them down into the cactus pose and to the sides. Instead of bringing

your elbows down to the sides, you squeeze the past behind you. The whole arm should look like chicken wings as you squeeze and hold before starting up the sequence again.

After you are done with this, you can bend a side bend with one arm up over your ear at a time. Just like the exercise in the last chapter. As you raise one of your arms over the side of the head towards the opposite side, bend to that side. Repeat on both sides five to seven times. Remember to link your breathing and to hold the seat of your chair with your free hand for balance.

Now, we can begin to use our dumbbells or whatever weight device you choose. Hold it in your right hand and lift the weight, bending the elbow and up towards your shoulder. When you bring the arm back down, point the elbow towards the side and then bring it up like that towards your shoulder. Keep alternating between the two directions as you lift and go down. Repeat these five to ten times on one side before switching to the other side. It does not matter how light the object you are using is, your body notices any extra weight and the motion will help build muscles and bone mass. Therefore, there is no reason to add more weight so you may feel like you are doing a workout.

Now, still using our weight we will start on the right arm again. Holding the dumbbell or whatever object you chose, lift your elbow to the side so that it is as high as your shoulder. Ensure the arm is bent at the elbow at a 90-degree angle. Now, lift the weight up, straighten your arms as if punching the arm and calm back down in the 90-degree bend. Repeat this five times.

There is another variation to this part of the sequence. What moment you bring the arm up into the bend you can move the arm across your body to the hip on the other side as if you are fastening your seat belt and then bring it up again and start over. If you decide to go this route, the same rules apply.

When you are done, switch to the other side and repeat.

Now back to our sitting posting, with legs hip width apart. Hold the weight in your right arm and let your arm rest to the sides. Hinge forward with your hips so that you are bent at a 45-degree angle. Keep your back straight. Now with the weight in your hands and fingers facing towards the chair, lift the wait up by bending the elbow so that it rises backward and above the line of your back. Repeat for five to ten times and switch to the other side. On the drop ensure that the arm is completely extended downward.

As you lift your elbow one last time, extend the arm out behind you. Bend the elbow and extend again. The elbow should be behind your back as you do this. Do these five to eight times and switch to the other side.

Still seated in the bent 45-degree angle and the weight in your hand. Flip your hands so that the fingers and palm are facing the back of the chair. In a wide arch,

swing the arms backward, always keeping it straight. Swing it as far back as you can and bring it back down to the level of your back line and lift it up again to as far back as you can. Repeat five to ten times before letting the arm down the lowest point and switching to the other side.

With the weight still in one of your hands, sit up straight with legs hip-width apart. Bring your elbows down towards your hips and swing your arms to the side while bend at a 90-degree angle, your elbows should be pointing at the hips all times. Swing the arms to the sides, so that they are as wide as the shoulder and then bring them back to the center sight in front of your stomach. Here, switch the weight from one hand to the other and repeat the motions again. Repeat these five to ten times. Remember to let your shoulders down when you do this.

After this as your arms reach the side, you can straighten the arm so as to point to the sides with your fists and then bend the elbow towards your hips again and then swing your hands to the middle to transfer the weight from one hand to the other and repeat the sequence. Do these five to ten times. Remember to always link your breathing, lifts with inhale and downs with exhales.

Now you can put the weight away and assume the starting seated position. Scoot over forward a little and hold your arms bent at the elbow in a 90-degree angle parallel to both your legs. I want you to open both your legs and the corresponding arm to the side at the same time while holding the 90-degree angle and then return to the center. Then do the same thing to the other leg and arm. Repeat the sequence five to eight times.

At this point you can incorporate the seated goddess pose, the warrior exercise and other torso and lower body exercises into the routine. After you close your eyes, take deep breaths to warm-down. That concludes the session.

KEY
TAKEAWAY

Don't be afraid to be creative when it comes to routines. It's a good idea to try all the exercises in the fourth chapter so you have a great idea of what works for you. Then you can incorporate those in any routine you find. If you want, you can make entire routines using the exercises that were shared in the fourth chapter. They will work.

Practicing routines regularly can help. The key is to be as consistent as you can be. To help with that, link the routine with another activity that you already do. For instance, if you normally go sit outside on the porch in the afternoon, maybe you could also do a 15 minute routine at the same time. That pairing will help with consistency and snoring, don't you forget.

Always start your yoga routine with a warm-up routine and end with a cool down routine. If you don't have the time, you can begin with breathing exercises shared in chapter two, but then proceed with caution especially if you are introducing more demanding exercises.

CONCLUSION

With the exercises in this book, you can be certain to regain strength, flexibility and balance that makes life worth living. It's not an overstatement since options for being active diminish while the benefits from being active do not.

You can use the exercises in chapter three at any time, and anywhere to help in that regard, if you can't find the time for a full quick session. You can also practice the routines in the last chapter for that purpose. Routines stick when they are piggybacked on another activity you already do. If you listen to podcasts in the morning, you can pair them with chair yoga sessions, for instance. Try to find those opportunities in your day when you can reliably do exercise and apply those. With enough repetition you should be able to do these often and with enjoyment.

You can always come back to the book to find exercises that apply to your situation that you can incorporate into your sessions. Exercises are just ingredients for a much larger workout.

My goal and aim is that you will benefit from the knowledge and encouragement in this book. Best wishes for your wellness! If you loved this book, please suggest it and write a review on Amazon.

Scan the QR Code To Leave a Review:

I wish you all the best and hope you have good health and happiness on the long journey ahead of you. Thank you for giving me the opportunity to share my expertise with you.

Baz Thompson

REFERENCES

Heron, M. (2021). National Vital Statistics Reports Deaths: Leading Causes for 2019. https://www.cdc.gov/nchs/data/nvsr/nvsr70/nvsr70-09-508.pdf

Jones, A. (2019, August 30). How to Correct 10 Common Mistakes People Make in Yoga. The Doctor Weighs In. https://thedoctorweighsin.com/how-to-correct-10-common-mistakes-people-make-in-yoga/#:~:text=%2010%20Common%20Mistakes%20People%20Make%20in%20Yoga

Mcgee, K. (2017). Chair yoga : sit, stretch, and strengthen your way to a happier, healthier you. William Morrow.

Pacheco, D. (2020, October 27). Physical Health and Sleep: How are They Connected? Sleep Foundation. https://www.sleepfoundation.org/physical-health#:~:text=%20The%20effects%20of%20sleep%20deprivation%20on%20physical

Pfau, W. (2016, August 25). How Long Can Retirees Expect To Live Once They Hit 65? Forbes. https://www.forbes.com/sites/wadepfau/2016/08/25/how-long-can-retirees-expect-to-live-once-they-hit-65/?sh=66f109466b4f

Southard, A. (2019, November 18). Why Breathing is Important in Yoga. Yoga Rove. https://yogarove.com/why-is-breathing-important-in-yoga/

Walker, M. (2019, January 29). How To Improve Your Sleep | Matthew Walker. Www.youtube.com. https://youtu.be/IRp5AC9W_F8

Webster, A. (2018, June 26). The Importance of Core Strength in Seniors. Elevating Seniors. https://www.elevatingseniors.com/core-strength-seniors/#:~:text=Core%20strength%20is%20important%20for%20people%20of%20all

www.ingramcontent.com/pod-product-compliance
Lightning Source LLC
Chambersburg PA
CBHW052117020426
42335CB00021B/2805